exercise your way to health:
type 2 diabetes

exercise plans to improve your life

dedication

For Phillip and Estelle

exercise your way to health:
type 2 diabetes

exercise plans to improve your life

Paula Coates & Thuvia Flannery

Diabetes
UK

The charity for
people with diabetes

Published in 2010 by
A & C Black Publishers Ltd
36 Soho Square, London W1D 3QY
www.acblack.com

ISBN 978 07136 8720 0

Acknowledgements
Cover photograph © Shutterstock
Inside photographs © Grant Pritchard, except 5, 12, 14, 19, 21, 25, 32, 35, 46, 57, 62, 66, 71, 88, 92, 94 Shutterstock and xii, 30, 59, 75 istockphoto.com
Illustrations by Jeff Edwards
Designed by James Watson
Commissioned by Charlotte Croft
Edited by Kate Turvey

This book is produced using paper that is made from wood grown in managed, sustainable forests. It is natural, renewable and recyclable. The logging and manufacturing processes conform to the environmental regulations of the country of origin.

Typeset in 9.25pt AGaramond on 12pt by Margaret Brain.

Printed and bound in China by WKT

contents

acknowledgements

Thuvia and I would like to thank everyone who has supported and helped us while we were writing this book, especially those who are close and those who are now with us in spirit. Finally a big thank you to Charlotte Croft and Kate Turvey at A&C Black, my models and Grant Pritchard for his photography.

foreword

Diabetes is an important and serious worldwide health problem currently affecting 6% of the population, and is rapidly increasing in prevalence. With obesity now reaching epidemic proportions, type 2 diabetes is being diagnosed at an ever-younger age, including during childhood. This book is a welcome addition to the body of literature that covers this important public health topic.

The book describes the distinction and similarities between different types of diabetes, the ways it may present and the tests used to confirm it. It gives a brief description of the treatments available and talks about future research. It goes on to explain the importance of good diabetes control to reduce the rate and severity of complications. The United Kingdom Prospective Diabetes Study (UKPDS) reported the association between poor glycaemic control and macro and microvascular complications. This study found that as the level of glycaemic control increases, so diabetes related complications decrease considerably.

This book is patient-orientated. The author is very aware of the difficulties the individual with diabetes faces in trying to balance control of their condition with the stresses of daily living. The book is empathetic to the needs of the reader, whilst offering practical advice.

Patient education regarding lifestyle advice, including detailed recommendations on diet and exercise, leading to weight reduction, and smoking cessation, is particularly well covered and offers clear, simple and achievable solutions. Patients with diabetes are encouraged by the author to take control of their condition and actively participate in its management. No amount of good advice from the diabetes specialist team will make a difference unless the patient and their specialist are working as one.

We hope that not only will you find this book enjoyable, but also a work of great practical value in your day-to-day life with diabetes.

Dr Natasha Thorogood MBBS, Specialist Registrar in Diabetes and Endocrinology
Dr Stephanie E Baldeweg MD FRCPI FRCP, Consultant Physician in Diabetes and Endocrinology
(University College London Hospitals)

endorsement

As a busy working GP and musculoskeletal specialist I can highly recommend this book as essential reading for patients and clinicians alike. This book is well researched, concise and up-to-date, and written by a first rate, highly experienced physiotherapist. It will give much needed and added support for patients diagnosed with Type 2 diabetes who want to do all they can to understand and manage their condition.

Dr Gregor McEwan MB BS, Dip. Sports Med. Lon.

preface

Advice and education in the management of many chronic conditions has been part of my professional life for the past 12 years, working as a physiotherapist in the NHS. Many of my patients have had other chronic conditions as well as their diabetes and successful treatment has included empowering them to continue managing their overall health and diabetes through self-management. However, the initial idea for this book was more personal, coming from my own family experience: I realised how badly my mother managed her diabetes and how basic information could easily help her manage things better. I knew much of the information and what the government's healthy living advice was, but realised this wasn't readily or easily available. I also became increasingly aware that I too would run the risk of becoming one of the expanding diabetic population by virtue of my family history and ethnicity. I wanted to find out what I could do to manage it if I did, or perhaps even delay or better still avoid it.

I know I can positively influence my own health and well-being, and in this book Paula and I will share with you the knowledge and experience we have gained.

Thuvia Flannery

introduction

This book is designed to help you understand your diabetes, what caused it, what treatments are available and how you can help yourself to manage your condition. It will explain why you should exercise and how that may interact with your medication. It also provides a step-by-step guide on how to exercise safely and how to measure your effectiveness and recognise your achievements. All these factors will allow you to take control of your personal situation and attain real and positive outcomes in your health and quality of life.

This book is split into three main parts.

Part 1 covers the basics that you need to know about your diabetes. It includes all the answers to the questions you wish you had asked when still with the doctor, but didn't ask because you were busy taking on board the fact that you had just been diagnosed. Once you know exactly what you are dealing with, it is much easier to manage and formulate a plan to move forward with your life.

Part 2 looks at what you can do to help yourself – the changes you can make to your lifestyle that will help you become fitter, healthier and in control of your own health. It is all too easy to feel out of control when you have been newly diagnosed and this book aims to give you back that control. In this part of the book we will guide you in both helping yourself and in explaining where to go and who to see when you need to seek medical advice.

Part 3 covers exercise, and how you can strengthen your body, lose weight and improve your overall health and fitness. Exercise has been shown to positively influence type 2 diabetes and to help reduce many of the risk factors associated with the condition. The exercises will show you how to get fit no matter how unfit you are now. This section also shows you how to monitor your own progress with simple tests that you can perform at home. When you see the results of adding exercise to your life, you will wish you had started sooner.

what can I do if I have type 2 diabetes?

People are generally living longer. Medical science has made huge advances in the treatment of many acute and chronic conditions and so contributed to extending our life expectancy. While there is as yet no cure for diabetes, it can therefore affect your health over a long period of time. Diabetes affects many people and can have a significant impact on lifestyle. So how can you manage such a condition which can profoundly affect your life, at home, work and play?

A diagnosis of diabetes may come out of the blue or it may be made over a prolonged period of time. Either way, once you are diagnosed it is easy to feel overwhelmed and perhaps that the condition has taken over you and your family's lives. The need to take medication on a daily basis and monitor your blood sugar levels daily can reinforce this feeling. It is important to understand that your condition can become a serious problem and specialist medical advice is always vitally important. However, there are some simple steps you can take to regain a sense of control over this situation and work proactively to improve the management of your diabetes, hand-in-hand with any prescribed medication, and so make a dramatic difference to your quality of life.

One method of taking control is active 'self-management'. When you take care of your body, it will take care of you, allowing you to enjoy life now and also prevent problems in the future. This book will show you how making changes yourself can lead to a happier and healthier you.

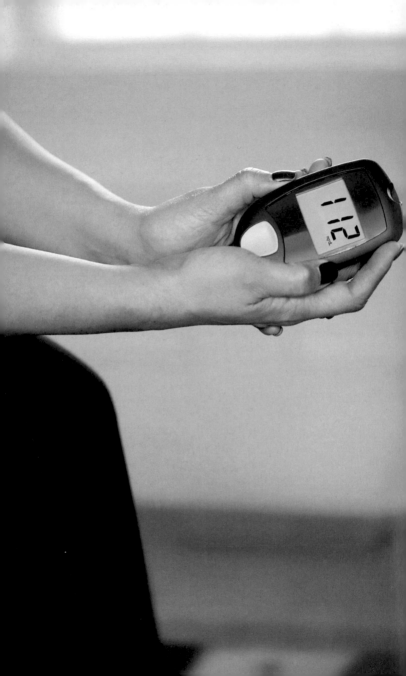

part 1

understanding diabetes

what is diabetes?

Diabetes is a condition in which too much sugar/glucose is found in the bloodstream. This usually occurs when there is not enough of a hormone called insulin available in the body or the insulin that is being produced does not work sufficiently well. Medically this condition of high blood sugar is known as 'hyperglycaemia' ('hyper' = high + 'glycaemia' = glucose).

Glucose is incredibly useful stuff, as it is the main fuel for the body's cells and is required in varying amounts, depending on the activity levels of each cell and your body as a whole. Insulin is produced in the pancreas and secreted directly into your bloodstream. It's also quite smart, as it allows the glucose in your blood to enter the cells of the body, giving them 'energy' and so allowing them to function.

Commonly, diabetes can occur if:

- little or no insulin is produced by the pancreas

- cells become resistant to the effects of the insulin produced

- the insulin produced does not work

- a combination of the above.

We are still not entirely sure what really causes diabetes. To make matters a little more complex there are three main types of diabetes to consider:

- type 1

- type 2

- gestational (may be referred to as type 3).

Other types of diabetes exist, including Maturity Onset Diabetes of the Young (MODY) and diabetes insipidus. These are discussed briefly later in the book.

type 1 diabetes

- This is also known as 'childhood', or Insulin Dependent Diabetes Mellitus (IDDM).

- It is rarely diagnosed in individuals over the age of 40.

- It is an autoimmune disease, i.e. where the body's defence systems malfunction and attack a specific type of cell in the body – in this case the insulin-producing 'beta' cells found in the pancreas.

- As a result little or no insulin is produced by the body, which causes the presence of high blood sugar or hyperglycaemia.

Between 5 and 15 per cent of the 2.3 million diabetic population in the UK have type 1 diabetes. That is some 115,000 to 345,000 individuals, men and women, boys and girls. Children with type 1 diabetes will grow up to be adults with type 1 diabetes as there is no way of preventing or curing the disease at present. Immediate treatment is essential, as undiagnosed or untreated type 1 diabetes can in some cases result in death. Type 1 diabetes cannot be managed without insulin. However, once a regular treatment regime has been developed people can generally lead a full and active life.

type 2 diabetes

- This was originally considered to be a disease of old age and was previously known as Non Insulin Dependent Diabetes Mellitus (NIDDM).

- Type 2 is now the most common form of diabetes, representing 85–95 per cent of people diagnosed.

- It is thought that up to 500,000 non-diagnosed cases may exist in the UK today.

- More and more people in developed and developing countries are being diagnosed, possibly because as people become more affluent their diets change, and they may be less active or have less time to exercise due to work commitments.

- More alarming is the increase in the diagnosis of children, some as young as seven years of age, with type 2. This is thought to be primarily due to increased levels of obesity and lower levels of physical activity.

Type 2 diabetes is considered by many in the medical profession to be in some respects a more complex condition to successfully manage once it is established. However, as you will find out in this book, it can be managed very well if caught early on and if you are informed, able and motivated. If that's the case, many sufferers require less prescription medication and in some cases no medication at all.

gestational diabetes

- This is often diagnosed in women during pregnancy when an abnormally elevated blood sugar level is detected.

- Gestational diabetes can affect 3–10 per cent of pregnancies and it is thought that the hormones released during pregnancy may lower the body's sensitivity to insulin, leading to high blood glucose.

- It is usually managed successfully during the pregnancy, but is associated with an increased risk of the mother developing type 2 diabetes after pregnancy.

- Delivery of a high birth weight or hypoglycaemic (low blood sugar) baby may also indicate gestational diabetes. The latter indicates that the baby is used to producing high amounts of insulin to cope with the mother's high blood sugar. After delivery it may take some time for the baby's system to adjust and so reduce its insulin production.

This book does not cover the management of gestational diabetes in relation to exercise. Specialist medical advice should be sought to avoid complications for both mother and child.

diabetes insipidus

Diabetes insipidus, which is much less common than diabetes mellitus, occurs when the complex system that regulates the amount and type of fluid within the body stops working properly. This happens when the anti-diuretic hormone (ADH) produced by the brain fails to prevent the kidneys from producing urine, either because not enough ADH is being produced, or because the body is responding to it incorrectly.

Although diabetes insipidus and diabetes mellitus share a name, the two conditions are almost totally unrelated. The symptoms of increased thirst and frequent urination are seen in both types of diabetes, but that is almost the only thing they have in common.

This book does not cover diabetes insipidus – for more information see www.diabetes.co.uk.

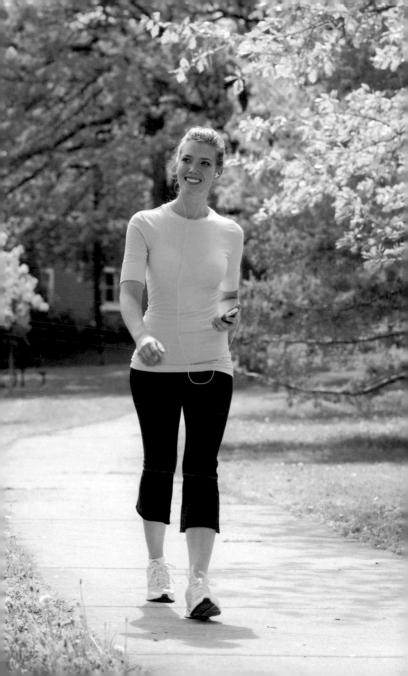

insulin and how it works

Insulin is the most important of the two hormones produced by the pancreas, whose role is to regulate blood glucose and therefore energy supply to cells. The second hormone is called glucagon.

insulin and glucagon

The amount of insulin and glucagon in circulation are dictated by:

- what type of food you have eaten, mainly carbohydrates
- how much exercise your muscles are doing
- how active your body cells are.

After you eat a meal, any kind of carbohydrate gets broken down into glucose and enters the bloodstream, causing your blood glucose to rise and insulin to be released by the beta cells in the pancreas. Insulin works by improving the uptake of glucose from the blood across cell membranes and into the individual cells of the body, rather like a key opening a door (see fig. 1.1). Once in the cell, the glucose is used as energy to fuel the various cellular activities that collectively allow the body to function healthily. The overall result is a drop in circulating blood glucose levels.

The pancreas detects the reduction in blood glucose and slows or stops the release of insulin. The cells now have the energy they need to function. Excess glucose is converted to glycogen (the name given to stored glucose) and stored in the liver and muscle, where it can be readily called upon in times of increased physical activity or cellular demand (during ill health, for example, or states of shock). The hormone glucagon, produced by the alpha cells in the pancreas, is secreted at such times to instruct the liver to release its stores of glucose into the bloodstream to meet the cells' energy demands.

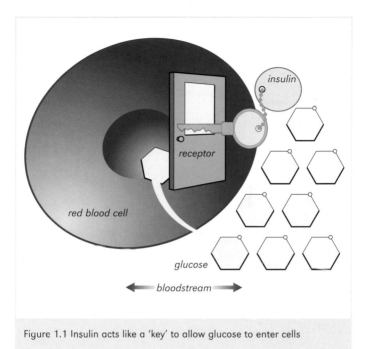

Figure 1.1 Insulin acts like a 'key' to allow glucose to enter cells

'Laughter is the best medicine – unless you're diabetic, then insulin comes pretty high on the list.'

Jasper Carrott

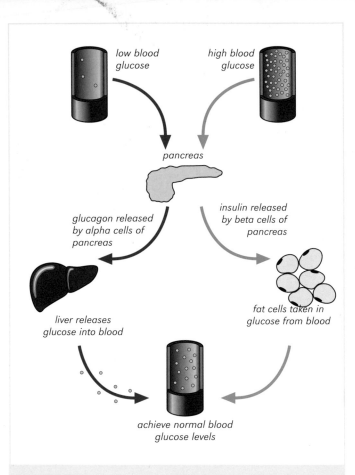

Figure 1.2 Normal, healthy control of blood glucose involving the balance between insulin and glucagon

signs and symptoms of diabetes

If the body produces too little insulin, or what there is does not work properly, glucose remains in the bloodstream, the cells are denied their fuel and the energy system breaks down. Excess blood glucose has to be removed by the body and the most obvious method is through increased urination. The early signs of diabetes are therefore often detected by finding glucose in the urine using a simple 'dip' test carried out by your nurse or GP. Other symptoms may be tiredness and unusual thirst, which are clearly associated with the loss of this energy-rich fluid. In severe cases, some people may also present with rapid weight loss. This occurs because the body starts to use alternative fuel sources, such as body fat, because the cells are starved of their primary fuel, glucose.

So the warning signs are:

- needing to urinate more than normal

- feeling thirsty all the time

- unexplained weight loss

- unexplained tiredness

- blurred vision

- altered sensation in your hands or feet.

These symptoms typically worsen over days to weeks.

In type 2 diabetes, the decreased sensitivity to insulin in those cells requiring energy causes hyperglycaemia and associated tiredness, as cells are not receiving adequate fuel and the body is unable to function normally. Unfortunately the increase in blood sugar generates more demand for insulin, the beta cells of the pancreas are unable to produce enough, and so the hyperglycaemia continues. The body tries to remove the excess glucose in the same way as before, through increased urination. However, with type 2 diabetes the signs and symptoms are likely to be much milder, and so possibly go unnoticed for longer.

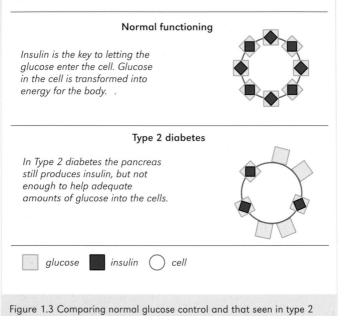

Normal functioning

Insulin is the key to letting the glucose enter the cell. Glucose in the cell is transformed into energy for the body.

Type 2 diabetes

In Type 2 diabetes the pancreas still produces insulin, but not enough to help adequate amounts of glucose into the cells.

glucose   insulin   cell

Figure 1.3 Comparing normal glucose control and that seen in type 2 diabetes

detecting type 2 diabetes

Type 2 diabetes is more likely to be detected:

- when you go for a general health screening or an operation
- in follow-up care after a heart attack or stroke
- when a wound isn't healing quickly, because of damage to blood vessels from high levels of blood sugar
- because you've given birth to a high weight baby or have a hypoglycaemic child (see page 20).

diagnosing diabetes

Getting tested and diagnosed early is the key to managing your diabetes effectively. Most people are diagnosed with diabetes after a simple blood test, referred to as a 'fasting' plasma glucose test. This looks at the amount of glucose in the liquid part of the blood (plasma). People are asked to fast for at least twelve hours before the test so that the levels are not overly influenced by what they have eaten. This is because blood glucose levels can be elevated for several hours after a meal, while they are generally at their lowest first thing in the morning before eating.

This test is measured by calculating how many millimoles of glucose are present per litre of blood (mmol/l) or milligrams per decilitre (mg/100 ml). Your blood sample usually has to be sent to the hospital laboratory to be processed, and you should expect to receive the result within seven days in most cases. Normal blood glucose ranges from between 4.0 and 6.0 mmol/l (90 mg/100 ml) with an average of 5.0, and this is the range that people with diabetes aim to achieve via medication and diet. A fasting glucose over 7.0 mmol/l (126 mg/100 ml) could indicate diabetes, as this is classed as hyperglycaemia (raised blood sugar).

fasting glucose test results
Two fasting glucose measures above 7.0 mmol/l are considered a positive diagnosis for diabetes. However, a positive result in the absence of clinical symptoms of diabetes could mean that you will need additional testing.

If the picture is still uncertain after a fasting blood plasma test then you may be asked to have further blood tests aimed at gaining a better picture of your blood sugar. This could be a repeat of the fasting test and/or random testing of your blood. The latter is done when a drop of blood, obtained from pricking your finger, is placed on a special testing strip and inserted into a glucose monitor, similar to that seen in Figure 1.4. This may be done at home or your GP's surgery, with the result being displayed by the monitor in seconds. This type of testing does not routinely involve fasting. A reading of 11.1 mmol/l (200 mg/ 100 ml) or greater would be deemed as hyperglycaemia (raised blood sugar) and strongly suggestive of diabetes.

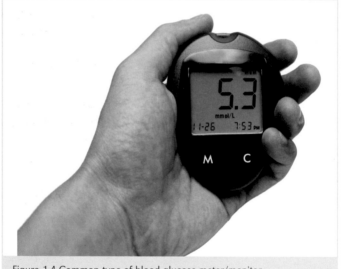

Figure 1.4 Common type of blood glucose meter/monitor

Your GP or health provider may also want to measure blood sugar by asking you to eat a specific amount of carbohydrate (75 g in the form of a sweet liquid), and then measure your plasma glucose two hours later. Readings of 8.0–11.1mmol/l would be diagnostic of diabetes indicating some failure to manage blood glucose normally. This test is referred to as a 'glucose loading test' and can be used to detect early diabetes. It is routinely used to test pregnant women suspected of suffering from gestational diabetes.

blood tests at a glance

- fasting glucose plasma test with a reading of 7.0 mmol/l (126 mg/100 ml)
- plasma glucose at or above 11.1 mmol/l (200 mg/100 ml) two hours after a 75 g oral glucose load, as in a glucose tolerance test
- repeated random plasma glucose at or above 11.1 mmol/l (200 mg/100 ml).

These levels will indicate problems with glucose control, and positive results together with other symptoms of diabetes almost certainly indicate a diagnosis of diabetes.

In the absence of obvious symptoms of diabetes, as discussed previously, it may take some time to make a firm diagnosis. The best advice is to attend every appointment or test that you are requested to, even if this interferes with work, childcare or other commitments. An early diagnosis is the next best thing to prevention. Early identification of diabetes often means that successful management may only involve changes in diet and activity levels. A later diagnosis may lead directly to medication to treat the diabetes and medical complications.

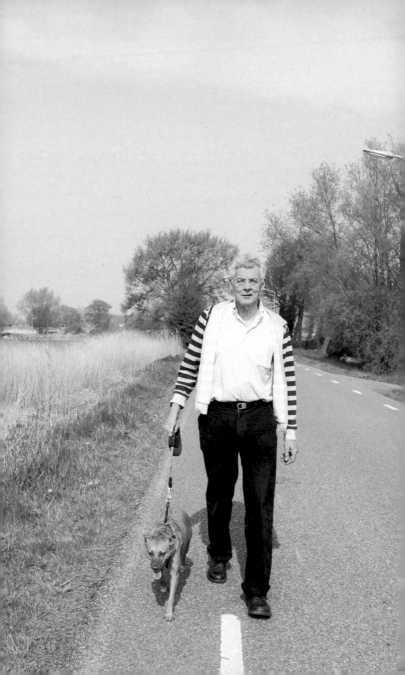

myths about diabetes

Like many other chronic diseases diabetes is subject to many common misconceptions. Some of these are listed below.

Myth: You can catch diabetes
Fact: This is not true. Diabetes is a condition that can affect many people due to family history, lifestyle and the presence of other common chronic conditions such as high blood pressure and high cholesterol.

Myth: You get it from eating too much sugar
Fact: This is not true. All forms of carbohydrate are converted into sugar (glucose) as part of normal digestion. However, eating foods that are high in sugar may lead to obesity, which in turn increases your risk of developing diabetes.

Myth: Type 2 diabetes is a mild form of diabetes
Fact: This is not the case. Diabetes is diabetes, and all types must be monitored and treated equally.

Myth: Diabetics eventually go blind
Fact: Although diabetes is the leading cause of blindness in people of working age in the UK, it is possible to limit its effects on eyesight by:

- regular eye tests
- controlling blood pressure and glucose levels
- giving up smoking
- keeping active
- watching your weight.

Myth: You can't drive if you're diabetic
Fact: Provided your diabetes is well controlled, there is no reason to suggest that you are less safe on the roads than any other driver.

Myth: People with diabetes can't do sport
Fact: Steve Redgrave, six-times Olympic Gold medallist, and ex-footballer Gary Mabbutt, would disagree.

Myth: Diabetics need special food
Fact: A general healthy diet low in fat, salt and sugar, but including fresh fruit, vegetables and starchy foods, eaten at regular mealtimes, is ideal.

pre-diabetic states

If you are told that you are pre-diabetic, this can mean one of two things:

- You have impaired fasting glycaemia (IFG) – people with fasting sugar levels between 6.1 and 7.0 mmol/l are considered to have IFG, which is associated with glucose intolerance and increased risk of cardiovascular disease. Glucose intolerance is where blood glucose levels remain above normal. Some studies have shown that IFG can progress into type 2 diabetes in as little as three years.

- You have impaired glucose tolerance (IGT) – people with plasma glucose at or above 7.8 mmol/l two hours after a 75 g oral glucose load are considered to have IGT, which is associated with 'insulin resistance'. Insulin resistance (IR) is the condition in which normal amounts of insulin are inadequate to produce a normal insulin response from fat, liver and muscle cells. This results in an increase in blood glucose and then insulin as the body tries to produce more insulin to remove the excess glucose. IGT carries an increased risk of cardiovascular problems and the likelihood of developing type 2 diabetes.

what is metabolic syndrome?

High plasma levels of insulin and glucose due to insulin resistance often lead to metabolic syndrome and type 2 diabetes. Metabolic syndrome is a collection of risk factors that increase the risk of cardiovascular disease and type 2 diabetes itself. It is not entirely clear how this occurs, but it results in damage to the internal walls of the arteries and causes them to narrow (atherosclerosis). High blood sugar secondary to insulin resistance does appear to be associated with this state.

Signs and symptoms of metabolic syndrome are:

- high blood pressure
- central obesity (fatty deposits primarily around the waist)
- elevated triglycerides ('unhealthy fats')
- increase in Low Density Lipoprotein (LDL) ('unhealthy/bad fat')
- decrease in High Density Lipoprotein (HDL) ('healthy fat').

There is more about triglycerides, LDL and HDL on page 20.

Of the two pre-diabetic states, IGT is more likely to develop into a full diabetes diagnosis and oral medication may be prescribed at this stage. However, this said, type 2 diabetes is usually caused because of lifestyle choices to eat too much and exercise too little.

how did I get diabetes?

Both type 1 and type 2 diabetes have a hereditary element, so if a member of your family has diabetes, you have an increased chance of developing it too.

risk factors for developing type 2 diabetes

Type 2 diabetes is thought to occur when a person has a collection of risk factors that can trigger the disease. It is therefore likely that the symptoms can be 'silent' until the disease is quite established.

Research has highlighted key risk factors, many of which can be directly influenced by you. Positive changes in lifestyle and regular screening could dramatically reduce your risk of developing diabetes.

- **Family history** – if a first degree relative, i.e. a parent or sibling, has type II diabetes, this increases your risk. Some studies have shown that if there is a history of diabetes in both parents, the child has a one in two chance of developing it.

- **Obesity** is probably the greatest risk factor. A Body Mass Index (BMI) of 30 or more (see page 40) is classed as obese. Even if you have a BMI of 27 this is also considered a risk. The exact level of risk varies according to ethnicity and age, but some experts suggest that a BMI of 30 or over would give you a tenfold increase in the risk of developing type 2 diabetes.

- **Ethnicity** – type 2 diabetes is more prevalent in south Asian (Pakistani/Indian), Afro-Caribbean and south Pacific peoples. Levels of type 2 diabetes are up to five times higher in the UK in Afro-Caribbean and Asian groups than in the Caucasian population.

- **Metabolic syndrome** – people with insulin resistance or impaired fasting glucose may also have elevated cholesterol and a higher risk of obesity.

- **Age** – the risk increases over the age of 45, with the greatest risk in the over 65 age group.

- **High blood pressure** – there appear to be two links here. First, people with high blood pressure are far more likely to have diabetes than people who have normal blood pressure. Secondly, if you have type 2 diabetes you have a tendency to develop high blood pressure,

obesity and risk

Black and white men with a waist measurement of over 37 inches (94 cm), Asian men with a waist measurement over 35 inches (89 cm) and women measuring over 31.5 inches (80 cm) are at risk. This 'apple shape' figure is particularly associated with the development of diabetes. Later in the book we will suggest ways to help you lose weight.

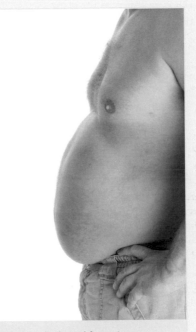

Figure 1.5 The apple-shaped figure is most at risk of developing type 2 diabetes

possibly through the mechanisms involved in insulin resistance and obesity which damage the lining of the blood vessels and lead to narrowing of the arteries. The combination of the two disease processes can increase the risks of coronary artery, vascular and kidney disease.

- **Elevated cholesterol** – cholesterol, a lipid (fat), is manufactured by the liver from the fatty foods that we eat, and plays a vital part in allowing the body to function normally. However, we have 'good' cholesterol, in the form of High Density Lipoproteins (HDL) and 'bad' cholesterol, in the form of Low Density Lipoprotein (LDL) and triglycerides. The trick is to get the right balance, otherwise they contribute to the clogging up of arteries and lead to poor circulation, heart attacks and strokes.

cholesterol

Blood cholesterol can range quite dramatically, however levels above 6.0 mmol/l are considered to be high and a risk factor for arterial disease. Government advice recommends a target cholesterol level of less than 5.0.

In the UK, two out of three adults have a total cholesterol level of 5.0 or above. In England, men, on average, have a level of 5.5, and women have a level of 5.6.

- **Lack of exercise or physical activity** can reduce your levels of good cholesterol (HDL). Regular exercise can help to reverse this and help maintain a healthy balance in your cholesterol in conjunction with a healthy diet.

- **Women with past gestational diabetes** – women who give birth to a child that weighed over 9 lb (4 kg) have been shown to have an increased risk of developing type 2 diabetes. Up to 40 per cent of women who had gestational diabetes go on to develop type 2 diabetes within 5 to 10 years of giving birth.

Other conditions with links to type 2 diabetes include:

- **Sedentary or inactive lifestyle** – this is often associated with being overweight. In pre-diabetic people who are obese, the risk of developing type 2 diabetes is higher.

- **Coronary artery disease** – because of damage to the lining of blood vessels.

- **Polycystic ovarian syndrome** (PCOS) – this affects up to 5 per cent of women and is a cause of infertility. Insulin resistance, type 2 diabetes and obesity are strongly associated with this condition, although the reason for this is unknown.

drug treatment

type 2 diabetes

If you have type 2 diabetes you will usually be prescribed tablets by your GP or other health provider. These need to be taken on a regular basis and you may need to take two or more different types. The two most commonly prescribed groups are biguanides and sulphonylureas.

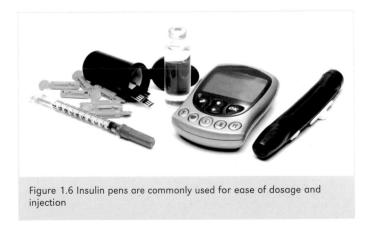

Figure 1.6 Insulin pens are commonly used for ease of dosage and injection

Biguanides work in two ways. They help to stop the liver producing new glucose and also overcome insulin resistance by making insulin carry glucose into muscle and fat cells more effectively. Metformin is the generic name for a common example of this type of drug – brand names include Glucophage and Fortamet.

> ## metformin
> Because Metformin has an effect on insulin resistance it is often given to people who are pre-diabetic and dangerously close to developing full type 2 diabetes. It is generally taken twice a day with meals but it may also be prescribed in a long-acting form that is taken once a day. In both cases the amount can be increased to obtain the best control over your blood sugar.
>
> Metformin can be passed on in breast milk so breast-feeding mothers cannot take it.

Side-effects of taking Metformin can include bloating, nausea and vomiting, and diarrhoea. These side-effects are thought to occur in one out of every three patients but are usually not severe enough to discontinue treatment. One in 20 people with severe symptoms may have to stop taking the drug or take a lower dose to reduce the side-effects.

Sulphonylureas are another group of drugs. These stimulate the pancreas to produce more insulin and also to help to make the insulin work more efficiently. Gliclazide is the generic name for a commonly prescribed example of these drugs – brand names may include Glucozide or Glizid.

gliclazide

Gliclazide, in tablet form, may be taken once a day before breakfast, and in some cases an evening dose (before food) may be added. Mild nausea and/or headaches can be common side-effects. Unfortunately this drug has been associated with weight gain and can occasionally cause hypoglycaemia (low blood sugar). The symptoms of low sugar could include faintness, disorientation and sweating. You should check your blood sugar using your glucose monitor, but usually a sweet biscuit (digestive type) should improve things.

If you are increasing your dose of this type of drug or have just started on it, you should ensure that you have regular mealtimes and a healthy snack (see page 54) to hand at all times. This is particularly important if you are away from home or work, driving or on public transport.

The above information is general and non-specific. It is not intended to tell you which medicine is right for you, and you should seek medical advice regarding your medication and any proposed changes to it.

changing from tablets to insulin

If you have had type 2 diabetes for a number of years you may find that tablets alone are no longer controlling your blood sugar. This can be part of the general ageing process. At this point, many people start using insulin injections, and may still take some tablets to manage their condition successfully. Starting on insulin does NOT mean you have developed type 1 diabetes, but simply that your type 2 diabetes is being treated differently.

additional medications
Other drug treatments exist for type 2 diabetes – to find out more you can visit www.diabetesuk.org. Some examples are:

- **prandial glucose regulator** – stimulates the pancreas to produce insulin; can only be taken at mealtimes.

- **thiazolidinedione** – has been used since the late 1990s and is a family of drugs that help to lower insulin resistance in cells, so that the existing insulin is more effective.

- **alpha glucosidsase inhibitor** – works by slowing down the absorption of starchy foods from the intestine, thereby slowing the rise in blood glucose after meals.

blood monitoring
Further blood testing may be required to check your blood sugar over a more prolonged period of time (4–12 weeks) to see how well medication or lifestyle changes are influencing your diabetes. This test is called the **glycosylated haemoglobin or HbA1c test.**

Red blood cells have a normal lifespan of 120 days. Glucose molecules join haemoglobin (the central part of the red cells) so forming glycosylated haemoglobin. Once joined, they cannot be separated until the death of that cell. In people with poorly controlled diabetes there is an increase in the level of glycosylated haemoglobins.

Normal healthy ranges are between 4 and 5.9 per cent. Levels above 7 per cent are seen as excessive and require rapid medical advice. A significant elevation of HbA1c can lead to diabetic complications such as eyesight problems or damage to the vessels of the kidney.

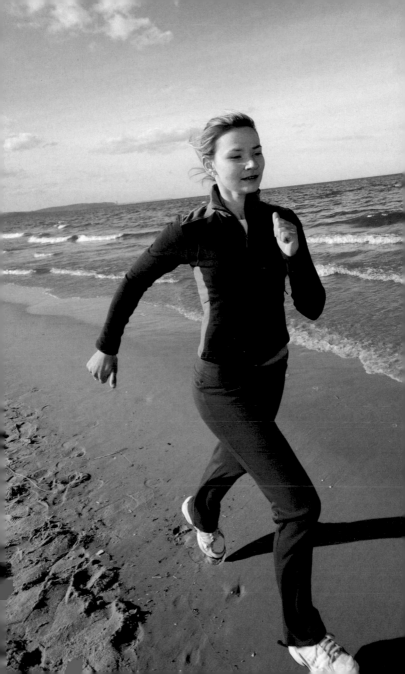

what's my prognosis?

After you've been diagnosed, the name of the game is to control your blood sugar as well as possible. However, we also know that weight and exercise play an important role in avoiding the complications of the disease such as obesity, high blood pressure and high cholesterol. To make it easier, this can be divided into good and bad control of blood sugar.

good control

Spotting type 2 diabetes or pre-diabetic states is crucial. If you have a positive result on any of the tests described above, the treatment options will be discussed between you and your health provider and will include:

- advice on how to control your diabetes by what you eat

- oral medication

- advice on exercise.

The earlier you know about type 2 diabetes, the better you can manage your condition and get a good outcome with a combination of the above treatments/advice.

'I had no idea that diabetes could affect so many aspects of your life and I found that hard. Once I had the reasons for this explained, more than once, I realised just what I could do to make things better today and for tomorrow.'

Paul, type 2 diabetic

poor control

acute complications

Type 2 diabetics are less likely to have such vast swings in levels of blood sugar than people with type 1 diabetes, as they are still producing some insulin; however, as the disease progresses, or if they become critically ill, this can become more of a reality for them too.

Complications include:

- **Diabetic ketoacidosis (DKA)**
  This is a dangerous and life-threatening condition that always requires emergency medical attention. If there is too little insulin, and therefore no metabolic access to glucose as fuel for cells, the liver resorts to metabolising fat into ketone bodies (fuel normally used for the brain). An elevation in these ketone bodies causes the blood pH to fall, making it acidic. A pH below 6.1 is incompatible with life. If untreated, DKA can lead to coma, and if the metabolic crisis is not corrected it may be fatal. This is more common in type 1 diabetes.

- **Hyperosmolar Non-Ketotic State (HONK)**
  The symptoms of HONK are similar to those of DKA; however, it has an entirely different cause and so requires different treatment. High blood glucose (greater than 16 mmol/l) causes water to move from the cells into the blood (via osmosis) which is then excreted by the kidneys. If left untreated this leads to dehydration and the loss of the chemicals (electrolytes) that help to balance body functions. This can lead to lethargy and eventual coma. This is more common in type 2 diabetes than type 1, because type 2 diabetics still produce some insulin and so the liver does not begin to metabolise fats, as it does in DKA.

- **Hypoglycaemia**
  Too much diabetic medication (insulin or tablets), insufficient food and/or excessive exercise, can cause blood glucose levels to fall too low. Symptoms include sweatiness, confusion and agitation. In

extreme cases this can result in coma, seizures and death. Prompt action is needed: anyone suffering a hypoglycaemic episode should immediately be given sugary foods or drink to correct their low blood sugar. In extreme cases hospitalisation and medical treatment may be needed.

Exercise induced hypoglycaemia can be a common occurrence with diabetes and so the following must be considered:

- When and for how long you exercise (insulin and dietary intake)
- The intensity of your program (how hard you work)
- Testing your blood sugar before, during and after exercise
- Always having a sugary drink or snack to hand to raise your blood glucose if necessary.

chronic complications

Poorly managed type 2 diabetes can lead to extensive long-term health problems. Chronic complications include:

- **Cardiovascular disease (CVD)**
  Chronically high blood sugar leads to damage to the small vessels (microvascular) and large arteries (macrovascular). This makes them weaker, more prone to damage and with a reduced ability to allow blood to flow through them. This encourages the deposit of fatty 'plaques', causing the blood vessels to narrow (atherosclerosis). If, for example, the blood vessels supplying the heart are affected (coronary artery disease), you may experience angina and have an increased risk of heart attacks. Diabetics have a fivefold increased risk of developing CVD compared to non-diabetics (www.diabetesuk.org).

- **Peripheral vascular disease (PVD)**
  As a result of CVD, over time tissues in the extremities do not receive enough blood, and you may have symptoms such as pain in the calves and legs on exercising or walking. The vessels supplying these areas will have narrowed, and without sufficient blood and nutrients tissues in these areas can become 'necrotic' (die) or become infected. Eventually it may be necessary to amputate the affected part(s). Individuals with poorly controlled diabetes represent one-third of all patients requiring some form of amputation in the UK.

- **Diabetic retinopathy**
  The growth of weak and poor quality new blood vessels in the eye, as well as swelling of the macula (the part of the eye that deals with the sharpness of image and colour sense) leads to poor vision and eventual loss of sight. Diabetes is the most common cause of sight loss in working age people in the UK.

- **Kidney disease**
  Damage to the kidneys due to cardiovascular disease can lead to chronic renal failure, which eventually requires dialysis (an external method of filtering blood to remove waste products). Poorly controlled diabetes is the most common cause of adult renal (kidney) failure in the developed world.

- **Diabetic neuropathy**
  Decreased or abnormal sensation, often beginning in the feet, may mean damage to the sensory nerves. If you are affected you may not be able to tell if you have injured yourself, and this can lead to ulcers or areas of infection (diabetic foot). Coupled with PVD and poor healing, this can result in the affected limb or toe being amputated.

- **Increased risk of stroke** – as a result of poor blood supply due to narrow and damaged blood vessels.

With the above in mind it is important that you have regular health screening to ensure that you are not affected by any of the above conditions. If you do have any of the above it may mean that you need to reassess with your diabetic specialist how best to continue exercising in a safe manner. The health benefits of exercise are still good for you, but may require modification.

Good control is obviously infinitely preferable to bad control. Poor control of your blood sugar causes damage to blood vessels that is often non repairable and degeneration to the eyesight that can't be reversed. Other significant health problems can appear that may restrict your life and cause early death.

This puts the ball firmly in your court! In the rest of the book we will look at ways you can make changes to your lifestyle that will help you control your diabetes and live a full and active life.

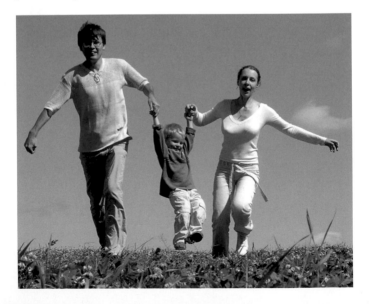

the cost of diabetes

There are currently 2.3 million registered diabetics in the United Kingdom. Government statistics for 2003 tell us that the management of this condition takes up 5 per cent of all the money spent by the NHS and is responsible for 9 per cent of hospital spending. That equates to approx £10 million per day to treat diabetes and diabetes-related problems. This is set to rise to 10 per cent of the NHS budget by 2011, according to Diabetes UK.

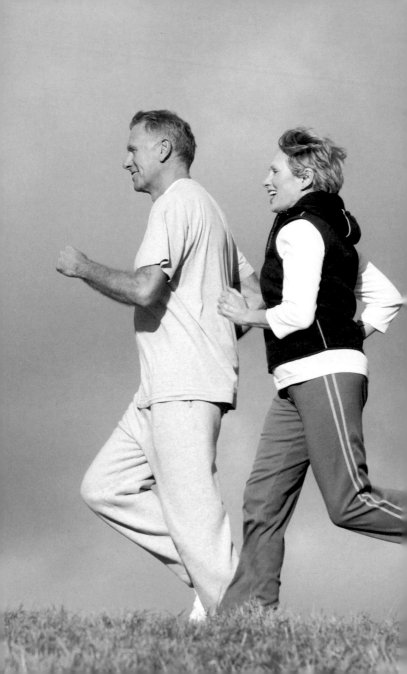

part 2

helping yourself to health

Now you know more about what diabetes is and how you may have developed it, it is time to learn more about how you can manage it. There are so many things you can do to make a real difference to how your diabetes impacts on your health and lifestyle. You can use the MOT questionnaire on pages 36–37 to help you think about your risk factors and then read on to learn how to minimise their impact on you and your diabetes.

where do I start?

You have already made a start by buying this book! The next thing to do is to take stock of your health and lifestyle. There may be obvious things that need to change, and this chapter will help you to identify others. By using the advice in this book you can find out how to manage your diabetes and improve your health.

> 'The thing with diabetes is there's nothing to see, no real symptoms at the beginning, so you just carry on as normal, don't you? It was only after my first heart attack that I really started to understand what was happening and what I should do!'
>
> Ray, 58, type 2 diabetic

Now for the good news! Type 2 diabetes, although a lifelong condition, can be managed very successfully and you as an individual can improve your glycaemic control and your overall health and sense of well-being. Being diagnosed with diabetes may feel like the end of something, but you can turn it into the beginning of a new healthy, motivated and vital you. Taking control allows you take responsibility for doing what it takes to manage your diabetes effectively. Your doctor can make treatment recommendations, but these won't make a difference unless you choose to follow them. He or she can't make decisions for you or make you change your behaviour. Only you can do that.

Remember, there is always more than one treatment option, as what works best for one person won't necessarily work best for you. Talking to your doctor about the different treatment options available will help you create and choose a plan that is right for you. Nobody knows more than you about your feelings, actions and how your diabetes affects you. This is why self-management is often seen as empowering – it puts you firmly back in control of your health.

how can I manage my diabetes?

All forms of diabetes share common themes in their management. Appropriate medication, a healthy diet, stopping smoking and regular exercise have all been shown to be beneficial. You may have no control over what kind of medication you have to take, but you can make changes to aspects of your lifestyle that will have a profoundly positive effect on your condition and make you healthier, happier and more energetic.

With type 2 diabetes there is a lot you can do to manage this condition, and in some cases prevent it developing. Let's start with a reminder of your risk factors for type 2 diabetes by answering the MOT questionnaire. How many of the risk factors (see box) apply to you, and have you ever thought you may be putting your health and diabetic control at risk? There are some factors you can't change, but it is important to be aware of what you can do to reduce your risk of developing diabetes and how to improve your control of the condition if you are already diabetic. The good news is that all the risk factors in green are the factors you can directly change.

risk factors
- family history of diabetes (parent or sibling)
- obesity
- ethnicity
- metabolic syndrome
- aged over 40 (Caucasians) or over 25 (Asians)
- high blood pressure
- high cholesterol
- sedentary lifestyle and minimal exercise
- smoker
- unhealthy diet
- heart disease
- polycystic ovary syndrome
- history of gestational diabetes during pregnancy.

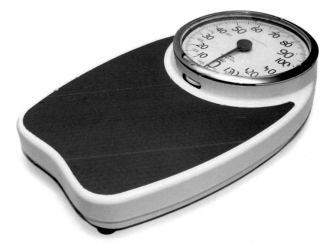

your personal MOT

Even if you have had diabetes for many years, it's worth stopping every now and again to take a look at your lifestyle to assess your current state of health and fitness. If you have been newly diagnosed then you definitely need to give some thought to your lifestyle choices so that you can avoid exacerbating your diabetic condition.

The MOT questionnaire is designed to give you a brief 'service history' and highlight the things that may have contributed to your developing type 2 diabetes or not allowing you to manage your blood sugar effectively. It is not designed to give you a full medical check-up. Only a professional can do that, so do consider a trip to your GP if you are worried about your blood sugar levels, struggling with your weight, or have other medical problems. Even if you are not diabetic but are worried about a family member or developing the condition yourself in the future, answering these questions will help you work out your risk factors and allow you to put a prevention plan in place. Remember type 1 diabetes does not have the same risk factors associated with its onset, but once diagnosed many of the above can profoundly influence your general health and lead to secondary diseases like heart disease and high blood pressure.

Your MOT will help you to focus on the here and now of your health – looking at problems that you may currently be dealing with and helping you spot the tell-tale signs of potential problems that may be lurking just around the corner. Answer the questions as honestly as you can and then count how many 'yes' and 'no' answers you have.

MOT questionnaire	yes	no
1 Would you describe yourself as unfit?		
2a Are you overweight or have you ever struggled with your weight in the past?		
2b Are you underweight?		
3 Are you a woman with a waist size of 31.5 inches (80 cm) or more, OR a black		

		yes	no
	or white man with a waist size of more than 37 inches (94 cm), OR an Asian man with a waist size of 35 inches (89 cm) or more?		
4	Are you currently on diabetic medication or have you had any recent changes to your medication in the last six months?		
5	Do you have any other diagnosed medical conditions?		
6	Do you have high blood pressure?		
7	Do you have high cholesterol?		
8	Do you smoke or have you ever smoked in the past?		
9	Do you have a sedentary lifestyle?		
10	Has exercise made your glycaemic control worse in the past?		
11	Do you drink more than your recommended weekly number of units of alcohol (14 units for women and 21 for men)?		
12	Does anyone in your immediate family have diabetes?		
13	Are you feeling constantly thirsty or going to the toilet a lot more than normal?		
14	Do you have a healthy and varied diet?		
15	Have you had your blood pressure and cholesterol levels checked in the past six months?		
16	Has exercise improved your glycaemic control in the past?		

How many 'yes' answers did you have to questions 1–13?

2–4 'yes' answers: SOME RISK OF TYPE 2 DIABETES
- You have highlighted some risk factors: read on to see what things you could change to improve your health and prevent yourself developing diabetes. See your GP if you have any symptoms that concern you.

4–8 'yes' answers: HIGH RISK OF TYPE 2 DIABETES
- You have a high risk of developing diabetes and if already diabetic could manage your blood sugar better. You need to consider making changes to your lifestyle to improve your health. You will be surprised just how quickly you see things improve.

8 or more 'yes' answers: VERY HIGH RISK OF TYPE 2 DIABETES
- You have highlighted many risk factors and may already have some symptoms related to diabetes. You must make changes to your lifestyle now to reduce your risk and improve your diabetic management. Keep reading and we will show you how. Small changes now will make a big difference and may prevent or delay the onset of diabetes.

As you can see the MOT test is most valuable in assessing your risk factors for developing type 2 diabetes, but shows too where you can make those essential lifestyle changes.

The more yes answers you have to these questions, the more risk factors you have for poor diabetic management or developing type 2 diabetes. However, if you answered yes to questions 14–16, these are the right answers!

yes to questions 1, 2a, 12 or 13:
If you think you are unfit and overweight, you probably are! 'Yes' answers to these questions put you at a greater risk of developing diabetes and may have contributed to causing yours, but the good news is that you can change things and by improving your fitness you will start to lose weight too. You have also highlighted some of the early

symptoms of diabetes and should see your GP for a check-up. To learn what your weight should be, see Figure 2.1. There are some great ways to improve your fitness: just turn to page 92 to see how to walk yourself to fitness and weight loss.

yes to question 2b:
Being underweight is just as bad for your health as being overweight. Many people think that being thin is better than being fat, but this is not always the case. It can be a sign that something is wrong and you are not as healthy as you could be. If you have started to lose weight recently it may be a sign of diabetes. As we saw earlier, this occurs because the body starts to use alternative fuel sources, such as body fat or muscle, because the cells in your body cannot get their primary fuel (glucose) from what you are eating.

yes to question 3:
If your waist size is equal to or higher than the figures shown you are at risk of developing type 2 diabetes. If you are already diabetic you must lose weight to improve the management of your diabetes. Research has shown that if you carry your excess weight around your waist you have a body type that puts you at a greater diabetic risk.

weight check

Take a look at Figure 2.1 and find your height at the side and your weight along the top or bottom. Follow a line across the chart from your height until you reach the line that corresponds to your weight. Are you the right weight for your height? If not, it is time to do something about it – even small changes to your lifestyle can help you achieve the right weight to improve your health. See the healthy eating advice on page 45 and the easy-to-follow exercise programme on pages 77–86.

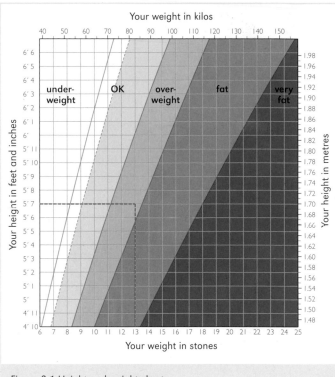

Figure 2.1 Height and weight chart

yes to question 4 and/or 5:

If you are already taking medication for your diabetes, it is important that you are also taking steps to improve your health and ensure your diabetes is well managed. This book will show you how and highlight areas that you may be able to improve. If you have any other medical condition for which you are taking medication, it is crucial that you try to improve your health. All medical conditions will see great improvement with simple changes to your lifestyle such as stopping smoking, eating healthily and making sure you exercise.

yes to question 6 and/or 7:

If you know you have high blood pressure or high cholesterol it is important to reduce both. Both conditions have a direct impact on your risk of developing diabetes and how well your diabetes is managed. Tables 2.1 and 2.2 show what your blood pressure and cholesterol levels should be. Your GP can test your blood pressure and cholesterol levels and if necessary give you tablets to help lower them. Stopping smoking, taking exercise and eating a healthy diet will all help reduce them too.

It is normal for cholesterol levels to be slightly higher in women, but there is some medical opinion to suggest that those at risk of heart disease should aim for even lower levels.

Blood lipid	Good	Borderline	High
Total cholesterol	5.0–5.6	6.0	6.5 and above
LDL cholesterol ('bad cholesterol')	2.0–3.0	4.0	4.5 and above

Table 2.1 Healthy and unhealthy cholesterol and triglyceride levels for people without heart disease (in mmol/l)

Blood pressure	Good	Normal	Borderline	High
Systolic (when the heart contracts and pumps blood out)	120 or less	120–130	131–140	141 and higher
Diastolic (between beats, as your heart fills with blood again)	80 or less	80–85	86–90	91 and higher

Table 2.2 Blood pressure levels for people without heart disease

yes to question 8:

If you smoke, now is the time to stop. There are 2000 deaths every week in the UK as a result of smoking-related diseases. Smoking has a direct causal link with peripheral vascular disease (narrowing of the arteries), will increase the risk of complications if you are already diabetic, and make you more likely to develop the condition if you are not. It's a no brainer! See page 56 for help and information on stopping smoking.

yes to question 9:

If you have a sedentary lifestyle or your job means you sit down for most of the day, it is even more important to make time to exercise. See part 3 for advice on lots of ways to exercise and how to become more active without even noticing. Just taking the stairs instead of the lift, or getting off the bus one stop earlier, will make a huge difference in a very short space of time.

yes to question 10 and/or 16:

If you have answered yes to either of these questions, well done, first of all for exercising. Research shows that exercise can reduce your diabetic risk by up to 64 per cent, and this is equally important for diabetics and non-diabetics. If you are diabetic you will have already realised how important it is to have a healthy and balanced diet to keep your sugar levels stable when you exercise. Experience will teach you how you need to adjust your diet as you start to exercise. One tip is to keep a healthy snack with you so you can quickly replenish your reserves after exercise. For advice on healthy snacks and menu ideas see pages 51–54.

Type 1 diabetics will require additional professional help in identifying a healthy diet that allows them to exercise regularly whilst limiting the risks of hypoglycaemia. Advice on what, how much and when to exercise, insulin and carbohydrates, should be sought from your GP or diabetic specialist prior to attempting an exercise programme.

yes to question 11:
If you drink a lot of alcohol you are adding sugar into your diet with no nutritional benefit at all. Most of us like a drink, but you should know your limits and what is a healthy balance. Excess alcohol is linked to many short-term and long-term health problems which will make your diabetic management more difficult. Regularly drinking more than the recommended number of units over a long period can lead to complications such as:

- certain types of cancer, especially breast cancer

- memory loss, brain damage or even dementia

- increased risk of heart disease and stroke

- liver disease, such as cirrhosis and liver cancer

- stomach damage

- weight gain.

Measure/type of drink		Alcohol by volume	No. of units
half pint of ordinary strength beer/lager/cider	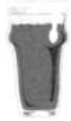	4%	1.1
330 ml bottle stronger beer	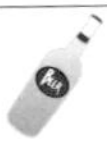	5%	1.7
small glass of wine (125 ml)	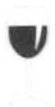	12–14%	1.5–1.75
large glass of wine (175 ml)	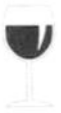	12–14%	2.1–2.45
single measure of spirits (25 ml)		40%	1

Figure 2.2 Units of alcohol per type of drink

Know how many units are in your favourite drinks (see fig. 2.2) and drink in moderation. For more information see www.drinkaware.co.uk.

yes to question 12:
In part 1 we looked at the increased risk of becoming diabetic if you have a family history of diabetes. The good news is that it is the best early warning you can have to reduce your risk factors and prevent diabetes in yourself and your family.

yes to question 13:
If you are needing to drink, feeling thirsty, or going to the toilet a lot more than normal, and you have other risk factors for diabetes, it is worth going to see your GP and ask if you can be tested for diabetes. In case you think this is wasting your and your doctor's time, it is worth knowing that diabetes is under-diagnosed and is much easier to treat and simpler to manage if diagnosed early. See page 11 to see how your doctor tests for diabetes.

yes to question 14:
Well done! Keep a check on both your blood pressure and your cholesterol levels. Tables 2.1 and 2.2 will show you whether your test results were borderline or high. If so, you will need to make some changes to make sure they come down. Stop smoking, don't drink excessive alcohol, and follow a healthy diet. If you haven't been tested, then ask your GP to test you now.

yes to question 15:
Well done! A healthy diet is so important for good health, to control your diabetes and reduce your diabetic risk. If you need advice on healthy eating see opposite.

Now you know your MOT results and your risk factors, it is time to find out how you can make changes to improve your health. Let's start by looking at healthy eating and exercise.

The benefits of exercise as a way of successfully managing your diabetes vary between type 1, type 2 and people with IGT (see page 16). Those with IGT are most responsive to regular exercise – it leads to an increased glucose uptake by the muscles.

Type 2 diabetics can also make significant improvements in glycaemic control with exercise, as well as benefitting from weight loss, decreased blood pressure and lower cholesterol. This can act as an 'insurance policy', not only improving health and well-being now, but also off-setting the age related changes that eventually effect us all.

healthy eating and diabetes

As a diabetic, eating a healthy balanced diet and making sure you don't feel thirsty is one of the most important things you can do. If you don't, you will soon start to feel the effects and will notice these more as you start to exercise. Imagine driving a car: you wouldn't dream of setting off on a journey without enough fuel.

Drinking enough is just as important as eating. Most people don't drink enough from day to day and function at a level of dehydration. If you feel thirsty, it's already too late: you are dehydrated. Your body needs 2–2.5 litres of fluid a day and when you exercise you will need more. The easiest way to keep a check on how hydrated you are is to monitor the colour of your urine. It should be a pale straw colour – any darker and you're already dehydrated.

'I hate taking tablets, so if the choice is between a lifetime of them and being careful about what I eat and staying active ... I'll do the latter!'
                    Maria, 43, with high risk factors for type 2 diabetes

Healthy eating can help you manage your weight and your blood sugar level and will improve how well you feel. It can also reduce your risk of developing heart disease, high blood pressure and high cholesterol.

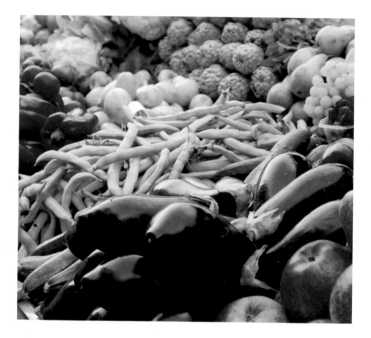

Healthy eating needn't be expensive – if you cook meals that use starchy foods and fruit and vegetables, aiming to eat less fat, salt and added sugar, it can actually work out much cheaper.

'I was diagnosed with diabetes when I was 42 and was told I could manage it by watching my diet alone. I didn't really know what that meant, but 20 years later and now on several types of medication, I do!'

Sheila, diabetic

what is a healthy diet?
A healthy diet contains:

- plenty of carbohydrates or starchy foods like bread, rice, pasta, breakfast cereals, potatoes and sweet potatoes – look for higher fibre versions where possible (like wholemeal bread or pasta)
- at least five portions of a variety of fruit and vegetables daily
- moderate amounts of dairy products (or alternatives if you don't tolerate them) – look for low fat versions where possible
- moderate amounts of protein, which is found in meat, fish, eggs, beans and lentils
- the occasional treat (foods that are higher in fat, salt or added sugar should only be eaten in moderation)
- minimal salt – always read the label.

why is healthy eating important for diabetics?
We all know that a healthy diet is important in maintaining a normal body weight and avoiding the problems associated with obesity. Diabetes is profoundly influenced by what you eat, your weight and how active you are. All these reasons make your diet more important when you are diabetic. This is why you need to be aware of what kinds of food you are putting into your body, not just to feed yourself but also as a way of keeping yourself healthy and less likely to become unwell. If you are unwell, even with a cough or cold, your diabetes can be affected. This is because you may find it more difficult to maintain good blood sugar levels when you are ill. For some reason it tends to make glycaemic control harder and blood sugars higher.

healthy eating and your child

Eating healthily yourself is one of the best ways to encourage your children to develop healthy eating habits and reduce their risk of developing diabetes in later life. Remember if you are diabetic, that counts as a risk factor for them becoming diabetic. Make sure their diet and weight don't also become risk factors for them.

As we have seen in part 1, most diabetic medication is aimed at lowering your blood sugar, so it is important to eat balanced healthy meals regularly to prevent your blood sugar from falling too low. Foods very high in sugar (sweets, cakes etc) should be limited or avoided, as they release their energy (glucose) into the bloodstream too readily. Wholegrain, high fibre foods tend to release their energy more slowly, so do not result in a dramatic increase in blood glucose after you digest them. This puts less strain on the pancreas to produce large amounts of insulin, and makes sure the insulin your pancreas can produce is effective in clearing the sugar from your bloodstream.

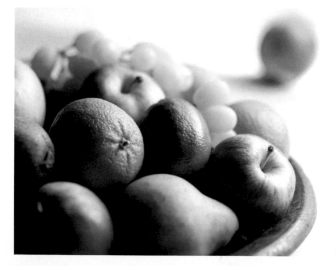

Figure 2.3 shows you the different food groups and how much of each should make up your daily meals.

Good quantities of fresh fruit and vegetables are the way forward. Heavily processed or pre-packaged food is not only generally high in sugar but also in salt and fat, all of which can contribute to weight problems, raise your cholesterol and raise your blood pressure. All of these factors will make managing your diabetes harder.

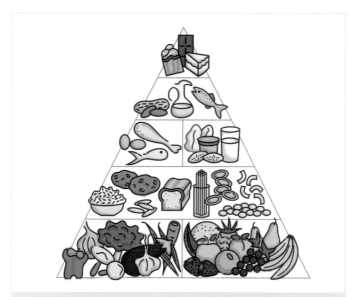

Figure 2.3 Balancing the food groups for a healthy diet

snacks

Always carry a 'healthy' snack such as fruit and a wholegrain bar with you to avoid the temptation to grab readily available chocolates and sweets when you're running late for lunch or on your way home from work. This is even more important when you are exercising.

the GI diet

In the past it was thought that all diabetics needed to be on a fairly restricted diet to manage their disease. We now know more about diabetes and realise that nearly all foods can be broken down into glucose, although some are broken down more readily than others. A popular diet which has proved helpful for diabetics is the GI diet, so-called because it rates foods by their glycaemic index. This means it measures the effects of certain carbohydrate foods on blood sugars after digestion. Foods with a high GI release glucose quickly into the bloodstream, thereby raising blood glucose dramatically. Low GI foods tend to release glucose more slowly and over a longer period of time. This is helpful for you as a diabetic, because it opens up a much wider range of foods and means you don't need a special diet.

Table 2.3 gives you an idea of where some foods sit in the glycaemic index scale. There are low, medium and high GI foods. No food is banned, but you just need to ensure that the majority of what you eat is in the 'low GI' group.

Classification	GI range	Examples
Low GI	55 or less	most fruits and vegetables (except potatoes and watermelon), grainy breads, pasta, legumes/pulses, basmati rice, milk
Medium GI	56–69	table sugar, croissant, brown rice, oranges, sweet potatoes
High GI	70 or more	cornflakes, baked potato, some white rices (e.g. jasmine), white breads

Table 2.3 Typical foods on the GI scale

Figure 2.4 compares high and low GI foods and how they affect blood glucose over time. You can see how high GI food (red line) causes your blood glucose to peak and slump quickly, in comparison to the low GI foods (blue line) which do not cause such extremes. The low GI menu suggestions below can help you keep your blood sugars following the blue line rather than the red one.

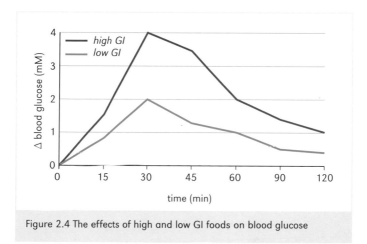

Figure 2.4 The effects of high and low GI foods on blood glucose

low GI menu suggestions

breakfast
- porridge (made with rolled oats)
- natural muesli
- All-Bran
- Special K
- wholemeal and mixed grain toast
- grapefruit.

lunch and dinner
Carbohydrates When you cook your meals you have better control over exactly what and how much salt, sugar and fat you put into them.

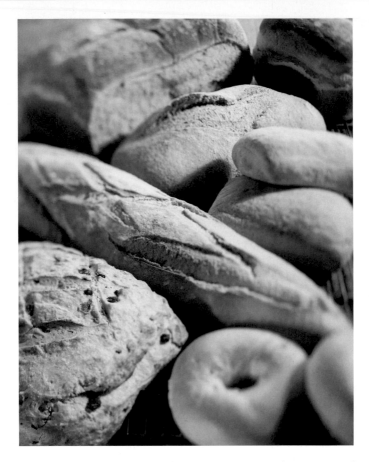

You can create delicious meat, fish and vegetarian meals using any of the staple low GI carbohydrates. You can also save money by using the leftovers for lunch the following day. Cooking your own meals is a better option than reaching for expensive pre-packed meals and sugar-laden fast foods. Use any of the following as the basis for a meal:

● wholewheat pasta
● new potatoes
● meat ravioli

- tortellini
- egg fettuccini
- brown rice
- white long grain rice
- pearl barley (this can be added to soups and stews)
- sweet potatoes (a nice change from the traditional potato)
- instant noodles/stir fry rice/pasta noodles (choose the ones from the fridge in your supermarket which don't contain added salt or sugar).

Low GI vegetables Cook vegetables in a hotpot, pasta bake, stir-fry, or soup, or simply serve with your favourite meat or fish. Making a salad for lunch is also a great way to get your five portions of fruit and vegetables a day. A good investment for your kitchen is a steamer. It cooks your vegetables to perfection and retains more nutrients than boiling them in water. Choose from:

- many types of frozen vegetables e.g. peas
- sweetcorn
- carrots
- aubergines
- broccoli
- cauliflower
- cabbage
- mushrooms
- tomatoes
- chillies
- lettuce
- green beans
- red peppers
- onions.

Low GI fruits Carry some dried fruit with you in case you feel peckish at work, and stick some pieces of fresh fruit in your bag to snack on during the day. You can even make a fruit salad or a smoothie and have it for breakfast – another great way to ensure you get your five-a-day.

All these fruits make a great snack or dessert:

- cherries
- plums
- grapefruit
- peaches (can be canned in natural juice)
- apples
- pears
- dried apricots
- grapes
- kiwi fruit
- oranges
- strawberries
- prunes.

Low GI sweets and snacks Replace that chocolate bar on the run or cream cake and biscuit with your cuppa with one of these healthy snacks instead. These will stop you having a sudden sugar high followed by a crash, and keep your blood sugars more stable:

- nut and seed muesli bar
- Nutella spread (on toast)
- hummus with carrot sticks
- peanuts (unsalted)
- walnuts
- cashew nuts
- nuts and raisins
- corn chips
- oatcakes
- rice cakes spread with peanut butter, hummus, or low fat cheese spread.

For more low and medium GI recipes and menu ideas see www.the-gi-diet.org and www.eatwell.gov.uk.

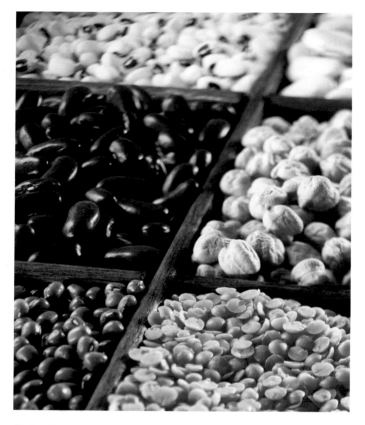

diabetic products
Leading diabetic charity Diabetes UK suggests that you avoid food marketed as being for diabetics for the following reasons:

- they are expensive
- they contain just as much fat and as many calories as ordinary products
- they can have a laxative effect
- they will still affect your blood glucose levels.

the truth about sugar free
Most people don't realise that most sugar-free products still contain carbohydrate and will make your blood sugar levels go up. Anything that contains starch or sugar, even naturally occurring sugar, contains carbohydrates.

Food containing the sweetener Sorbitol can have a laxative effect if you take too much. Some people report mild to severe diarrhoea and bloating.

If you require more information or advice on diet and diabetes, contact your GP who can put you in touch with a dietician. Alternatively, websites such as www.diabetesuk.org can give you more helpful hints on how to develop a healthy, balanced and 'sociable' diet that will be good not only for you, but for other members of your family too.

stopping smoking

Now you have read about the changes you can make to your diet, the next important thing to improve your health is to stop smoking. We all know the dangers linked to smoking and for you as a diabetic it really is crucial. If you need to be reminded about why you should give up smoking, read on.

Smoking causes numerous diseases and health problems, and not just for the smoker. Both smokers and non-smokers can develop smoking-related disease. For this reason, smoking is now banned in public places and a wide range of support services has been developed to help you quit smoking. If you are diabetic or have high risk factors to develop diabetes you really should stop smoking.

reasons to quit

People give up smoking for many reasons, from wanting to improve their health, to saving money, or reducing any potential harm to the health of their families. In the UK one person dies from a smoking-related disease every four minutes. If you are already diabetic, you have

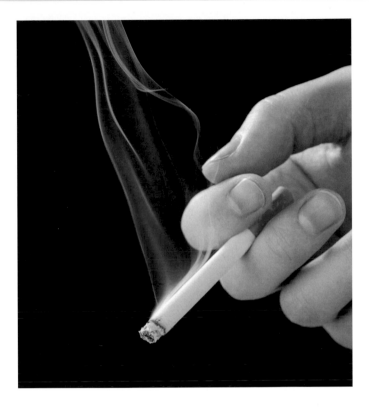

a greater risk of developing heart disease, high blood pressure and peripheral vascular disease (PVD); smoking increases this risk further and in turn will make controlling your diabetes much more difficult. If that is not enough to persuade you, take a look at this list of the other diseases that are caused by smoking and which will make your diabetes worse:

- lung cancer (smoking causes over 80 per cent of all lung cancer deaths)
- heart disease
- bronchitis
- strokes

- stomach ulcers
- leukaemia
- gangrene
- other cancers e.g. mouth and throat cancer.

Smoking can also make having a cold, chest problems and allergies like hay fever much worse, as well as increasing the number of wrinkles on your face and causing bad breath. It can make you cough and feel short of breath when you exercise. As we have already seen, feeling unwell makes controlling your diabetes much more difficult.

As well as improving your own health dramatically, here are some of the other advantages of stopping smoking:

- **It will boost your sex appeal:** it's a myth that smoking helps you lose weight – in fact it can cause cellulite. And kissing someone with a mouth like an ashtray is just plain revolting. Many ex-smokers find that their sense of smell and taste improves when they quit smoking. This is a perfect side-effect for enjoying your healthy new diet!

- **You will save money:** calculate how much you spend on cigarettes each week and multiply this by 52. Work out just how much smoking is costing you every year and you might be surprised how much you could save or what you could buy instead. How about a new car or a holiday?

- **You will protect your family's health:** breathing in other people's cigarette smoke can also cause cancer. If you are having second thoughts about giving up smoking for yourself, think about the people around you. Children exposed to secondhand smoke are twice as likely to get chest problems and more likely to get ear and throat infections and asthma. Smoking during pregnancy can affect both you and your baby's health, and if you are pregnant and breathing secondhand smoke you can pass on harmful chemicals to your baby.

types of treatment

When willpower alone is not enough, there are various treatments and plenty of support services to help you kick the habit. Many chemists offer a 'stop smoking' service and can advise you on the products available to help you quit. There are many types of treatment available. Some of the nicotine replacement therapy treatments are:

- **Nicotine gum:** When you chew nicotine gum the nicotine is absorbed through the lining of the mouth.

- **Nicotine patches:** Nicotine patches work well for most regular smokers and can be worn round the clock (24 hour patches) or just during the day (16 hour patches).

- **Microtabs:** These are small tablets containing nicotine which dissolve quickly under your tongue.

- **Lozenges:** Lozenges are sucked slowly to release the nicotine and take about 20–30 minutes to dissolve.

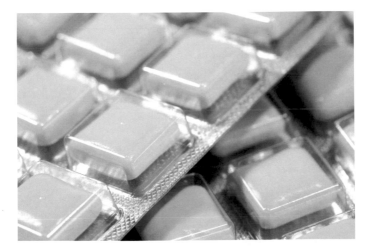

- **Inhalators:** Inhalators look like a plastic cigarette. The inhalator releases nicotine vapour which gets absorbed through your mouth and throat. This is a good option if you miss the 'hand to mouth' aspect of smoking.

- **Nasal spray:** The spray gives a dose of nicotine through the lining of your nose.

Other drugs that can help you to stop smoking are:

- **Zyban (Bupropion hydrochloride)**
  Zyban is a treatment which changes the way your body responds to nicotine. You start taking it one or two weeks before you quit and then for a couple of months to help you through the withdrawal cravings. It is only available on prescription from your GP and you cannot use it if you are pregnant.

- **Champix (Varenicline)**
  Champix works by reducing your craving for a cigarette and by reducing the effects you feel if you do have a cigarette. You start taking the tablets one or two weeks before you decide to stop smoking. Treatment normally lasts for 12 weeks. Like Zyban it is only available on prescription from your GP and cannot be used if you are pregnant.

helpful contacts

Smokers are four times more likely to quit by using the NHS Stop Smoking Services together with nicotine replacement therapy than they are by using willpower alone. Find your nearest NHS service by:

- visiting the NHS Smokefree website (http://smokefree.nhs.uk) for England and Wales or Smokeline (www.clearingtheairscotland.com) in Scotland

- texting GIVE UP and your full postcode to 88088

- telephoning the NHS Smoking Helpline (0800 022 4332) in England and Wales or Smokeline (0800 84 84 84) in Scotland

- asking your GP or pharmacist.

The NHS Smoking Helpline in England and Wales offers free practical advice about giving up smoking, as well as a free information pack, while in Scotland, Smokeline provides free confidential advice and support. Both Smokefree and Smokeline offer an 'Ask an Expert' service.

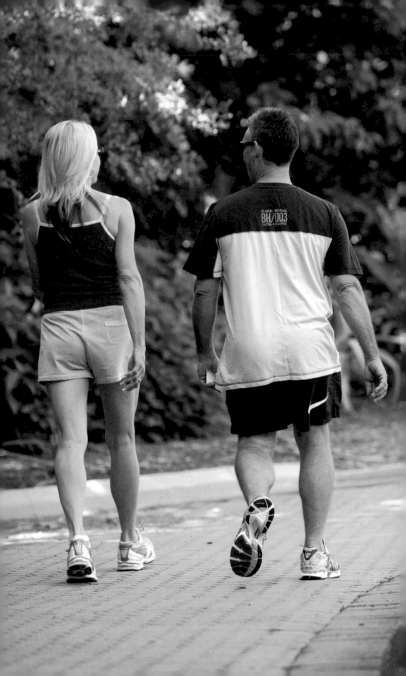

part 3

the exercises

what can exercise do for me?

When you've just been diagnosed with diabetes, perhaps the last thing to enter your mind is the concept of exercising! However, exercise has been shown to positively influence diabetes and also help reduce many of the risk factors for developing diabetes and associated with diabetes. Is it as simple as that? Yes it is!

The key to success is to find ways of getting more active and exercising in a way that is realistic for you. This doesn't always have to mean going to the gym or taking up sport – many people find it suits them better to go for a regular walk. Take a friend with you and use it as a chance to chat and catch up. Another great way to exercise and socialise is by joining a dance class. If you're looking for love, you could find that too while learning to dance! Introducing exercise into your life may be as simple as taking the stairs instead of the lift, or getting off the bus one stop before your destination – these small changes will help increase your basic fitness and gently introduce your body to the idea of exercise.

If you have never exercised before, you will benefit from the 'steady beginnings' section on page 74. This will give you a gentle programme to start with so you don't do too much too soon and risk a hypoglycaemic episode or injure yourself. If you have exercised before but perhaps have only recently been diagnosed as diabetic, or have just started or changed your medication, you will also benefit from reading this section. Even as an experienced diabetic you will benefit from a change to your usual routine. Read on and see if there is anything that can help you on a daily basis or with lifestyle changes.

> 'I just feel so much better when I exercise regularly and my blood sugar readings are better too! My advice is don't wait – get on with your diet and exercise now!'
>
> Ron, 50, type 2 diabetic

how much to exercise?
- Recent medical studies have shown that a short daily workout lasting 20 to 30 minutes is beneficial to health.
- Three or four sessions of 20-30 minutes of activity a week will be enough to have general health benefits and improve your fitness.
- Increase sessions to 60 minutes to help you lose weight and stop weight going back on.

Regular physical exercise reduces the risk of developing some of the leading causes of illness and death in the UK, as well as managing your diabetes. It can also help improve your mood and manage stress more effectively. For the greatest overall benefits, it is recommended that you do 20 to 30 minutes of aerobic activity three or more times a week and some type of muscle strengthening activity as well as stretching twice a week. If you are unable to do this, you can still gain substantial benefits by accumulating 30 minutes of moderate intensity exercise (see below) every day. Little and often will still make a difference.

Exercise can help you to:

- reduce the risk of dying prematurely from heart disease

- reduce the risk of developing diabetes

- reduce the risk of developing high blood pressure

- reduce high blood pressure if you already have it

- reduce feelings of depression and anxiety

- control your weight

- build and maintain healthy bones, muscles and joints

- improve balance and reduce the risk of falling.

'When you really think about it, it's easy! A normal but healthy diet and regular exercise can help to prevent all kinds of other diseases, so if it helps with your diabetic control too, well you'd be a fool to ignore that!'

Mandy, 45, pre-diabetic

how much should I do?

The aim of exercise is to achieve a beneficial level of fitness and health, both physically and mentally. How much you do will change as you become fitter and feel you can do more. There are different intensities of exercise: light, moderate and vigorous.

- **Light exercise** generally allows you to talk at the same time. Examples of light exercise include going for a walk, doing some light housework, or gardening.

- **Moderate exercise** should make you feel slightly out of breath. Examples of moderate exercise are going for a brisk walk, dancing, or walking up a hill.

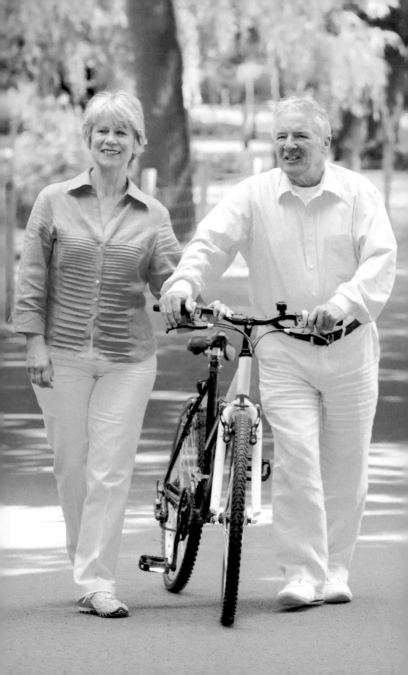

- **Vigorous exercise** should make you breathe rapidly, and you should feel as if you are just at the point where you are pushing your body's boundaries. Jogging, cycling, dancing, swimming and weight training are all vigorous forms of exercise.

What may be vigorous exercise for one person can be light exercise for another and vice versa. This means that just about anyone can exercise with the right motivation and guidance. The important thing is to take that first step and get started.

an unfit nation
Only 20 per cent of people in the UK get enough exercise to maintain a healthy lifestyle and satisfactory fitness level. The main reason given for not taking part in enough exercise is lack of time.

Exercise and physical activity can play a very important role in helping you control your blood sugar levels better. Before you start to make any changes to your lifestyle just take a moment to complete this physical activity readiness questionnaire. This checks that there are no major reasons why you shouldn't take up exercise.

It is important that you complete this questionnaire honestly before becoming more physically active.

Physical activity readiness questionnaire	yes	no
1 Has your doctor ever said that you have a *heart condition* and that you should only do physical activity recommended by a doctor?		
2 Do you ever feel *pain* in your chest when you do physical activity?		

		yes	no
3	Have you ever had chest pain when you are not doing physical activity?		
4	Do you ever feel *faint or have spells of dizziness?*		
5	Do you have a *joint problem* (also back problem) that could be made worse by exercise?		
6	Have you ever been told that you have high blood pressure?		
7	Do you have breathing problems?		
8	Do you have any problems with your liver, thyroid, kidneys or have diabetes?		
9	Are you currently taking any *medication*? If so, what?_____ Reason_____		
10	Are you pregnant, have you had a baby in the last 6 months, or do you plan to have a baby this year?		
11	Has your mother or father had any heart problems?		
12	Is there any other reason why you should not participate in physical activity? If so, what?_____		
14	Do you have a healthy and varied diet?		
15	Have you had your blood pressure and cholesterol levels checked in the past six months?		
16	Has exercise improved your glycaemic control in the past?		

YES to one or more questions:
If you answer yes to one of more of these questions or do not know the answer, you should discuss becoming more physically active with a member of your diabetes care team (doctor or specialist nurse) either in person or on the phone BEFORE starting exercise.

It is likely that you will be able to do the exercises you want to, you will just have to start slowly and build up. Just check with your care team first.

NO to all questions:
If you answered no to all of these questions it looks like you should be ok to exercise without too many problems. If you do have any questions about whether you are ok to start exercise speak with your doctor.

before you start

hypoglycaemia: are you prepared?
Exercise can help to improve glycaemic control, possibly leading to a reduction in oral medication in the case of type 2 diabetes. However, it can work so well at bringing down your blood sugar that you need to make sure it doesn't drop too low. You will need to time any exercise to fit in with your medication or insulin schedule, but you should also be prepared to deal with hypoglycaemia if it occurs.

- **Know the signs** – confusion, shaking, lightheadedness, or difficulty speaking, all indicate that you should stop exercising immediately.
- **Have a snack handy** – when your blood sugar is too low, you can quickly bring it back up with a low-fat, high-carb snack, such as jelly beans, a small bottle of non-diet soft drink (diet varieties won't contain the sugar you need), or fruit juice.

- **Exercise with a friend** – try to walk or work out with someone who knows that you're diabetic and who could help out in an emergency.
- **Carry identification** – even if you're just taking a walk around the local park, carry ID with your name, address and phone number, along with the dosages of your medication or insulin. Diabetic alert bracelets are available.

set your exercise goals

It's always helpful to have a goal – it helps keep you motivated, and makes you think twice about skipping an exercise session! What goal could be better than controlling your diabetes and improving your health? You may want to reach a certain weight, fit into a certain outfit, run 5 kilometres for charity – choose a goal that is right for you and go for it! It is also important to consider which forms of exercise will suit you. Exercising in several different ways can stop you getting bored, which can be an important factor during and after potential 'glitches' in your diabetic control. There are plenty of suggestions in this section to get you started, and alternatives to keep you motivated. Key points to remember are:

- An exercise class is a great way to keep you motivated and find an exercise partner. Most classes will have people of mixed ability, so you are bound to find someone at a similar level to yourself. Check for classes advertised at your local gym or in the local newspaper.

- Pick a date to start exercising and stick to it. Attending a salsa class every week is a great place to start and establishes a routine for you.

- Be realistic about the goals you set for yourself.

- If you are an experienced exerciser look at increasing the amount of training you are doing – it is important for you to be as realistic as a complete beginner.

- Overdoing things may cause problems with your glycaemic control and lead to hypoglycaemic episodes (see page 69), so don't do too much too soon.

- Even when you feel at your fittest, pace yourself and don't do too much. Problems and 'hypos' can arise at any time and may become an issue if you don't monitor how much you are doing generally and exercise wise.

- Stress and deadlines at work, moving house and gardening are all things that can impact on activity levels without you realising till it is too late.

- Don't aim too high and risk the disappointment of failure, or so low that the exercise has little effect and presents no challenge or personal achievement.

get the right footwear

Getting the right pair of trainers is one of the most important things you should do when you start to exercise. Diabetes can cause complications with the sensation in your feet: it is common to cut or blister your feet as a diabetic and not feel it as a result of damage to the nerves. This, combined with the potential for poor wound healing, means that it is extremely important for all diabetics, newly diagnosed or otherwise, to get sound advice and assessment regarding footwear. Prevention is definitely better than cure!

You can get advice about this and about your foot type – the shape of your foot and your arch – through your chiropodist or podiatrist. There are different types of trainers for different types of feet and a good trainer shop can help you get the right shoes for you. If you think you have any biomechanical anomalies, such as flat feet, see a podiatrist for an assessment (all have specialist training in diabetes management) before you start exercising, as there are insoles and appliances available which can make things much easier for you.

check with your doctor

If you have any other medical conditions as well as diabetes, it doesn't mean you can't exercise. However, it is important that you check with your doctor that you are not going to do yourself any harm.

- Most medical conditions will benefit from exercise, whether they are related to your mental or physical health. You may just need to be monitored until your level of fitness improves.

- Walking on a treadmill is helpful if you are new to exercise or have cardiac problems – training indoors can be safer as there will always be people around when you start to exercise, and you can stop whenever you like without having to worry about getting back home or to where you started.

- If you are taking medication for your diabetes and/or thyroid problems, you may need to monitor and adjust the amount you need when you exercise. If you have any concerns chat to your doctor.

illness, coughs and colds

If you are currently having a period of less well-controlled glycaemia, which can happen when you are ill, run down, or suffering from a cough or cold, wait until you are feeling better before you start a new exercise programme.

- After a cold it is important to return to exercise slowly. Your immune system will still be recovering, so take it easy to avoid getting another infection.

- With diabetes, any kind of infection can make it difficult to get good glucose control. You should monitor your blood sugars closely with a glucose monitor and contact your GP if you are struggling to get on an even keel.

pregnancy, exercise and diabetes

If you are pregnant and have been diagnosed with gestational diabetes you may still be able to exercise, but you need to check with your health provider or GP/midwife to see what is advisable for you.

After delivery and when you are ready, exercise is an excellent and obvious way to get your fitness back and decrease your chances of developing type 2 diabetes, and also have fun with your baby! There are many post-natal classes available: speak to your midwife or check to see what is happening in your area. For ideas of ways to exercise with your baby have a look at www.salsababies.co.uk and www.buggyfit.co.uk.

It is also important to make sure your tummy muscles are recovering and that you are doing your pelvic floor exercises. A good bra is even more important at this time. If you are breastfeeding your size will fluctuate, which makes getting a well-fitting bra difficult. Get measured for a sports bra from a good department store or specialist bra shop, and try to get measured when your breasts are at their fullest. A second 'pull over' soft bra or sports top with a built in bra/crop top will provide more support, and allow for any fluctuation in size.

exercise is for all

Exercise is available to everyone whatever their level of fitness, budget or lifestyle. It doesn't have to hurt and it can be fun. It comes in many flavours – you just need to choose your favourite. Once you know your abilities you can achieve your goals.

steady beginnings

The exercises that follow are intended to help those new to exercise, and those with more than six 'yes' answers on their MOT questionnaire. There are three exercise sections to choose from: a home workout programme, a swimming programme and a walking programme.

If you have been inactive for a while, you need to make a start with less strenuous activities such as walking or swimming. There is a walking plan on page 92, a swimming plan on page 89 and a section on exercising at home on page 76. Beginning at a slow pace will allow you to become fitter without straining yourself. As you become fitter, you will be able to do more.

All the exercises are designed to improve your cardiovascular fitness, that is, the health of your heart and your circulation. This will also improve your lung function. This kind of exercise is also called aerobic exercise, and uses all the main muscle groups in your body over a sustained period of time, increasing your heart rate to 50 per cent or more of its maximum level. To achieve a base level of fitness you can do anything you fancy that gets you outside in the fresh air and moving your body. Make the world around you your gym so you get the added bonus of fresh air!

> ### light intensity exercise
> When you are exercising and raising your heart rate it is normal to feel warm and slightly out of breath, but you should still be able to talk. To find the right pace for you, use some of your favourite music and sing along as you exercise.

However, if you need to exercise because of a medical condition such as diabetes, your GP can actually prescribe exercise for you! This makes it much more affordable if you would prefer to use a gym, and also makes sure that you have the advice and guidance you need. Most sports centres will offer exercise on prescription and have fitness instructors who are trained to understand your exercise needs. All you need to do is ask at your local sports centre and then discuss the prescription with your GP.

exercise at home

When you are exercising at home, make sure you clear a space, and put on comfortable clothes. This will make you feel more prepared for what you are about to do and less likely to put your feet up in front of the TV! Try putting on your favourite CD or radio station – music is a great motivator and singing along will help keep your breathing steady. You could even move out into the garden in the summer, though if you're worried about being seen by the neighbours, opening the window will be enough to keep you cool.

You may be surprised by how much exercise you can do at home, and it doesn't mean you need to build an extension for your own gym or buy expensive gym equipment. Look in your kitchen cupboards to find cans of beans or soup which are great to use as hand weights. If you do want to invest in exercise equipment, there are some fold-away exercise bikes and cross-trainers available on the market which won't take up too much space in your front room. Pedalling your way through the news or your favourite soap is a good habit to get into and keeps you motivated and in a routine. Argos, your local department store, Amazon and eBay may have some good value deals on exercise equipment too.

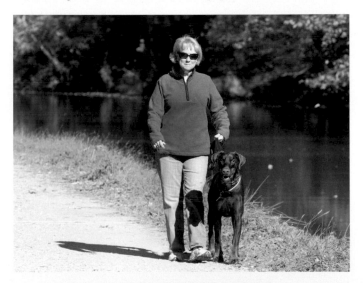

circulation exercises

If your diabetes is causing problems with your circulation or you have ulcers on your legs, exercise will help improve both. If you can't exercise for any reason, try these simple circulation exercises (known as Buerger-Allen exercises) which are usually taught to patients with peripheral vascular disease or PVD (see page 29). As a diabetic you can benefit too, especially if you are showing the early signs of PVD or have diabetic ulcers. These exercises need to be repeated 6 times at each sitting and work best if you can fit them in several times a day. They are easy to do and don't really feel like exercise.

- Sit on a bed or sofa with your legs supported and stretched out in front of you. Place your legs in an elevated position, on pillows, cushions, or even the arm or back of the sofa. Aim to have your ankles higher than your heart.

- Keep your legs in this position for 1–3 minutes, or until you see your legs blanching or whitening.

- Actively flex and point your ankles throughout.

- Then sit up with your feet on the floor for 2–5 minutes, or as long as it takes for the circulation and colour to return to your legs. The total time should not exceed 5 minutes.

- Place your legs in a horizontal position for 3 minutes before you repeat the process again 6 times.

The purpose of these exercises is to assist circulation in the legs when the blood vessels are compromised by atherosclerosis, vascular disease or diabetes. It will certainly help with the healing of diabetic ulcers on the lower leg.

'I wish someone had explained to me earlier all the problems that diabetes can bring if you don't look after yourself! I'm in my fifties now and some damage is already done, but I exercise, watch what I eat and have regular check-ups. I want to be around to play with my grandkids!'

Ann, type 2 diabetic

beginner's routine

This simple routine will build up noticeable pace and stamina in only a few weeks. Give it a go, and you will be enjoying exercise before you know it! Try doing this routine (steps 1–9) 3 times a week, and you will be impressed with your results. Once this becomes easy, progress to the swimming or walking programme (pages 89 and 92) and see your fitness improve even more.

warm-up and stretching

march on the spot

1 March on the spot for 2–6 minutes to warm up. Start at a moderate pace that you can maintain for the full 2–6 minutes. Swing your arms and lift your knees high. You should aim to become breathless but still be able to talk easily.

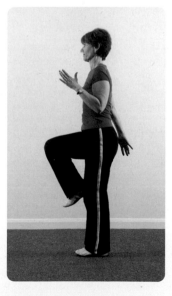

- week 1: march for 2 minutes
- week 2: march for 4 minutes
- week 3: march for 6 minutes

squats

2 Stand with your feet hip distance apart and your hands on your hips. Squat as if to sit down, and then stand tall, reaching one arm above your head. Lift your arms alternately and feel the stretch in your side. Aim to do between 5 and 15 repetitions.

- week 1: sit to stand 5 times
- week 2: sit to stand 10 times
- week 3: sit to stand 15 times

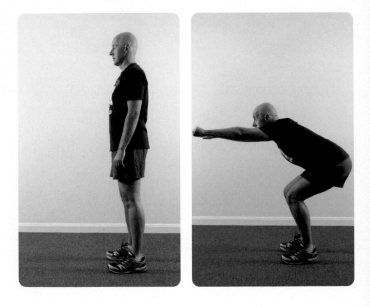

step back lunges

3 Stand with your feet hip distance apart and your hands on your hips. Step back with one leg, as far as you would if you were walking backwards, and then return it to the starting position. Repeat 5–15 times, holding the final step back and keeping your heel on the floor. Hold for 30 seconds, and then repeat with the other leg. You will feel the stretch in the back of your leg.

- week 1: step back 5 times
- week 2: step back 10 times
- week 3: step back 15 times

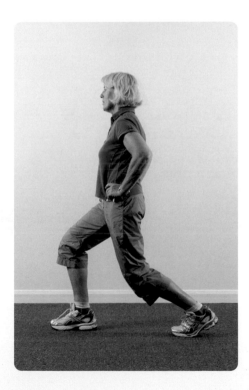

aerobic exercises

step-ups

4 Step-ups can be performed on a small box or at the bottom of your staircase. Step up and down with one leg 5–15 times and then change legs. This is one set. Continue for 2 to 6 sets with one minute's rest between each set. Maintain a good posture throughout by standing up tall with your shoulders back, looking straight ahead. Keep sipping water between sets so you do not dehydrate.

- week 1: step up 5 times for 2 sets
- week 2: step up 10 times for 4 sets
- week 3: step up 15 times for 6 sets

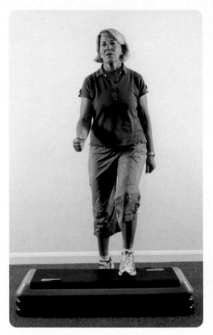

Safety point
If you have some altered sensation in your feet or eyesight problems, make sure that you can do this exercise safely. It would be best to use a low, well-lit step with an easily reachable banister.

bicep curl and press

5 Strengthening your arms with bicep curls and an overhead press is simple and functional. Hold a weight in each hand (see box), starting with 0.4–2 kg weights depending on your level of fitness. Stand tall and alternate your arms, bending your arm from your side to your shoulder, then pushing the weight above your head. Repeat 5–15 times for one set. Continue for 2 to 4 sets with a minute's rest between sets.

- week 1: lift 5 times for 2 sets
- week 2: lift 10 times for 3 sets
- week 3: lift 15 times for 4 sets

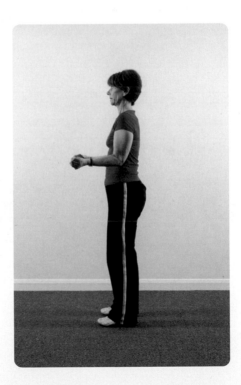

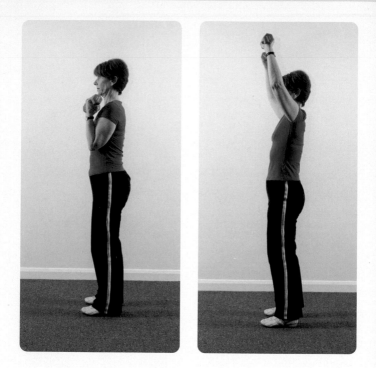

weights
You don't have to buy expensive weights: you can use tins of beans (400 g) or bags of sugar (1 kg) as weights in each hand. If you want to buy weights, start with light weights and progress as you become stronger. You can buy beginner's sets of 1–5 kg weights from most sports stores, but don't try to lift too much too soon.

side bends

6 Using your home-made weights in each hand, keep your arms by your sides. Slowly lean over to the right, allowing your hand to reach your mid-thigh. Allow the other arm to reach up and curl over your head. Repeat 5–15 times and then repeat on the left side. After one minute's rest, continue for 2 to 6 sets.

- week 1: bend to each side 5 times for 2 sets
- week 2: bend to each side 10 times for 4 sets
- week 3: bend to each side 15 times for 6 sets

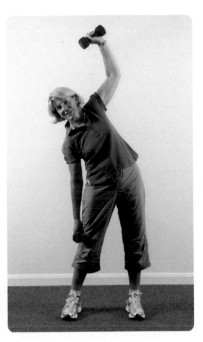

safety point
You may need to start this exercise without the weights if you have problems with your balance as a result of altered sensation in your feet.

winding down and stretches

7 March on the spot slowly for 2–6 minutes, concentrating on your posture and lifting your knees. Breathe deeply in and out, keeping your hands on your waist. This will allow your heart rate to return to normal as you keep moving, yet allow your body to cool down gradually.

- week 1: march for 2 minutes
- week 2: march for 4 minutes
- week 3: march for 6 minutes

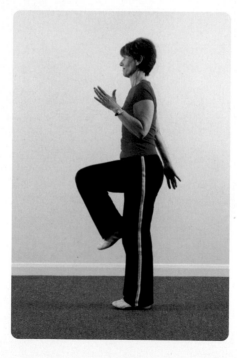

8 Stand with your hands resting on a kitchen surface or the back of a chair. Lift one leg out behind you and lift the foot off the floor. Squeeze your bottom as you lift and make sure you don't arch your spine. Repeat 5–15 times, and then change legs.

- week 1: lift each leg back 5 times
- week 2: lift each leg back 10 times
- week 3: lift each leg back 15 times

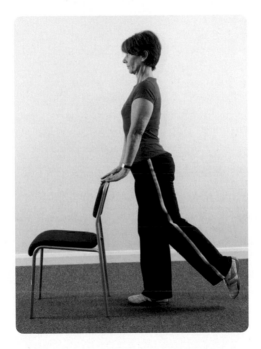

safety point
Again make sure that you have made the area as safe as you can – standing on one leg can be harder than you think if your balance has been affected by your diabetes.

9 While standing, take six deep breaths in through your nose. Breathe out through your mouth, making sure you empty your lungs. Gently pull in your lower tummy as you do this and feel your core muscles working.

> ### check your feet!
> At the beginning and end of every exercise session you should take a few minutes to check the condition of your feet. Look specifically for any areas of broken skin, chafing or rubbing that may have occurred as a result of exercising. If you do spot any areas of concern contact your GP or nurse straight away to have it assessed.

swimming

Your local swimming pool is a great place to start exercising if you have diabetes. If you're overweight, haven't exercised for a while, or have joint pain, balance problems, or foot pain from nerve damage, all of which are common problems with diabetes, the swimming pool is a great place to get active. Your weight is 'reduced' by up to 90 per cent in water and swimming can give you the buoyancy you need to keep exercising aerobically for longer than you may be able to manage on dry land. This is a bonus if you need to lose weight. Swimming is an excellent way to increase your heart rate, with an added benefit over walking as it exercises both the upper and lower body at the same time.

As with any new exercise, you must monitor the effects on your blood sugar and take the necessary action to control your diabetes. Always have a snack with you to eat after exercise in order to regulate your sugar levels.

aqua aerobics

An aqua aerobics class may be the best way to get a full-body workout, and you don't even need to know how to swim. Like any aerobics class, upbeat music and being with a group of people can make exercising more enjoyable and keep you motivated! Before choosing a class, make sure it is appropriate to your level of fitness and ability. Go and watch a class before you attend.

before you start

Here are some points to consider before you begin a swimming programme:

- **Always check with your doctor first.** He or she can help you identify the best options for you and particularly how to deal with any negative effects.

- **Is the pool easy to access and clean?** If you have loss of sensation in your feet how difficult is it to get in/out of the pool? Are the surrounding walking surfaces clean and even to avoid undue injury or infection?

- **Be extra-alert for low blood sugar symptoms.** It may be harder when you're in a pool to tell if you're sweating or feeling weak so you need to be more aware and get out of the pool as soon as you suspect a problem. If your blood sugar drops while you're in the water, you may not have time to get out and go to your locker to reach your snack, so keep a high-carbohydrate snack in a plastic bag on the poolside while you swim.

- **Talk to the lifeguard or your aqua aerobics instructor** and explain that you are diabetic. They will be able to monitor you and keep glucose tablets or a snack handy.

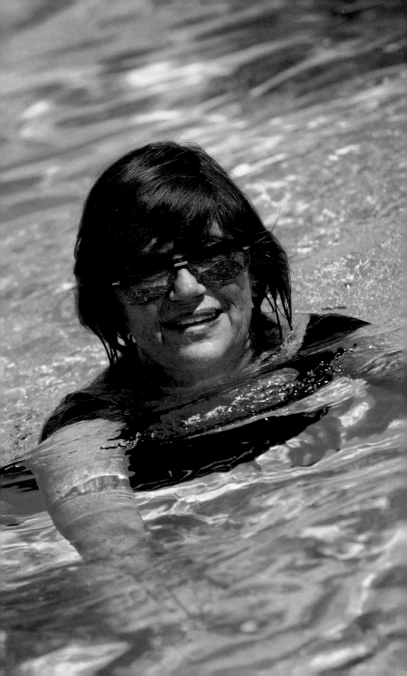

- **Protect wounds while in the water**. Swimming when you have an open wound or an ulcer isn't a good idea because it increases your risk of infection. Rather than missing your swimming session when you have a skin wound, ask your doctor or diabetic clinic whether a waterproof dressing is appropriate for you. Be sure to clear the use of a waterproof dressing with the pool manager before you jump in!

- **Protect your feet in water**. Diabetes can make your skin prone to slower healing, and serious infections in the feet can even lead to amputation in the most extreme cases. Wearing water shoes or aqua socks when you're swimming in the sea will help prevent cuts and injuries from rocks or other debris. Wearing protection in swimming pools is a good idea too, as the concrete floors or cracked tiles of some pools can be abrasive or sharp.

- **Glasses or goggles?** As a diabetic you may have problems with your eyesight. If so, ask when your pool offers times set aside for lane swimming. Swimming in lanes that are roped off and free from people splashing around will make things easier. Having your own designated lane reduces the chances that you'll collide with someone you couldn't see coming.

- **Shower immediately after swimming**. The chlorine from swimming pool water can dry out your skin and might cause it to crack, which will make you more vulnerable to infection.

- **Apply water-resistant sunscreen when you swim outside**. The water may feel cool against your skin, but you could still get sunburnt. Sunburn is not healthy for anyone, but it's particularly bad if you have diabetes because it can take longer to heal and, if it's severe, could raise your blood sugar level.

your swimming programme
To improve your aerobic fitness steadily, aim to swim two to three times a week.

weeks 1–2

Start by swimming twice in the first two weeks, say on Monday and Friday or Tuesday and Thursday, so that you have a day or two to rest in between. Aim to stay in the pool for about 30 minutes. Swim one length of the pool at your own pace, and then rest for one minute or until your breath returns. Swim 10 lengths.

weeks 3–4

You have already started to make swimming part of your weekly routine, and you can change the days if you need to, but make sure you still swim twice a week. Now think about adding an extra five lengths to each swim. Continue to rest for up to one minute after each length. You will be surprised how quickly you can swim this new distance. You may be in the pool more than 30 minutes when you first increase your number of lengths, but I guarantee that by the end of week four you will be swimming 15 lengths in 30 minutes. Now there's a goal for you! If, as you get fitter, you feel up to swimming two lengths before you need to rest, give it a try. If you are swimming with a friend, see who can finish first. The last to finish brings the healthy after-swim snack next session!

weeks 5–6

This is the time to increase your swimming to two lengths, if you haven't done so already, before resting for a minute. In week six, swim four lengths before taking your minute's rest. You will still swim 15 lengths, but now you are pushing your fitness and increasing the number of lengths you swim in each set. If you are swimming with a friend you can chat as you swim, and spend quality time while getting fit.

weeks 7–8

Now you have an established routine it is time to build things up a little. Introduce more lengths and increase the number of lengths in each swim set before you take that well-earned minute's rest. Swim five lengths now before you rest, and aim to swim 20 lengths in total. Try swimming a different stroke for each length – this will stop you getting bored and also use different muscles. See how much further you can swim without needing a rest once you increase your fitness.

weeks 9–10
Now you should be noticing changes in your fitness and your waistline! You are ready to progress and introducing a float can vary your lengths and make you train your arms and legs harder. Most pools will have floats that you can use – just ask the lifeguard. This is also a great way to improve your cardiovascular fitness. Hold onto a float with both hands and propel yourself through the water by only kicking your legs. Aim for five lengths before you take your minute's rest. It may sound like an easy option, but if you give it a go your legs won't agree, as they are doing all the work without help from your arms! For the next five lengths swim again, and then repeat the two sets.

weeks 11–12
Another way to use your float is to hold it between your knees and swim using just your arms to pull you through the water. Swim your regular set of five lengths, alternating with five lengths with the float between your knees. You may need to take rests, so take them as you need them – you will soon be increasing the number of lengths you can swim with just your arms as you get stronger. To have a mixed workout over the week, vary your programme each day. One day just swim, one day swim with the float in your hands, and one day alternate all three options – a length swimming, a length swimming with legs only and a length with arms only. Mixing it up will stop you from getting bored!

when to swim

Choose a time of day which suits you but make sure you have eaten and have some water with you to keep you hydrated. Don't exercise for at least two hours after eating, as this will make you feel nauseous. Make sure you sip water during exercise but don't drink too much – it is more important to drink regularly throughout the day to avoid dehydration rather than too much all in one go.

taking it outdoors: walking

As we have already said, you don't need expensive gym membership and you don't even have to get hot and sweaty to improve your fitness. Walking is not a soft option: you can actually burn more calories walking than running, if you vary your walking speed and style.

Exercise does not have to involve a complex regime. Current health agency advice includes trying to achieve 10,000 steps a day as a form of regular exercise. This makes it easier to incorporate exercise into your everyday life. Don't worry about counting every step, as a simple and inexpensive device that clips onto your belt/waist, called a pedometer, can measure it for you. To make a start, you can walk more simply by getting off the bus or tube one stop early, or buying your lunch from a shop further away from work. You will get fitter without really noticing!

Walking is an excellent way to ease into exercise if you have diabetes. It is a low-impact exercise and gets you out in the fresh air; but best of all it is easily accessible and free. Making a start is the first step. Follow the simple programme on page 93 and watch your fitness improve in six weeks. Try to maintain a good posture from head to toe and stride out so you can keep an even pace. Swinging the arms helps speed up your pace, and to progress as you get fitter you can swing your arms while holding weights.

Once you have built up your walking, it can be a good idea to progress to a mixed speed programme, where you mix periods of brisk walking with periods of slow walking, gradually increasing the duration of the brisk walk and decreasing the frequency of the slow walk. Try this after you have tried the walking programme I have outlined below. This allows the body to adapt gradually to the stresses of exercise and helps you to avoid injury.

Always take a small nutritious snack with you just in case you go a bit further than you intended or start to feel a little unsteady (the symptoms of hypoglycaemia). It may also be worth having some form of identity bracelet that clearly states you are diabetic and what type you have. This is only in cases of emergency when you are unable to verify that for yourself.

walk safe
It is important when starting a walking plan that you walk on routes that are safe. This includes walking at times of the day when it is light and where places are busy and not secluded if you plan to walk on your own. You can even leave a note at home with the time you left for your walk, where you are going and when you are due home. Take your mobile phone with you so you are always in contact.

your walking programme
This simple routine will build up visible pace and stamina in only a few weeks.

weeks 1–2
Start by walking every day. This may be as simple as walking to the station, getting off the bus one stop early or walking to buy your lunch. Taking the stairs instead of the lift also counts as walking and may be possible more than once a day.

weeks 3–4
You have already added walking into your routine without taking up any extra time in weeks one and two. Now think about adding an extra 15 minute walk into each day. This may be part of your route to work, to the shops or to a friend's home for coffee. You could offer to walk a neighbour's dog or give a new mother a break by taking her baby for a walk.

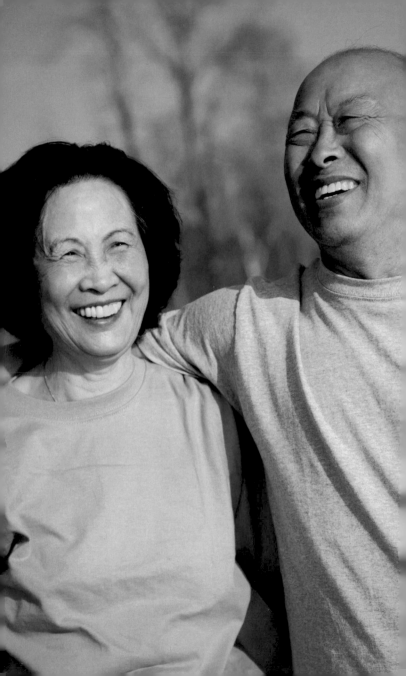

weeks 5–6

Increase your daily walking time to 20 minutes in week five and 30 minutes in week six. You can use this time to switch off and have time to yourself, or if you prefer, make phone calls and catch up with all those friends you never get round to calling back. Better still get a friend to walk with you and spend quality time while walking.

weeks 7–8

Now you have an established routine of daily walking, it is time to speed things up a little. Swing your arms and focus on striding out as you walk. See how much further you can walk once you increase your pace. A pedometer will help you monitor your distance. Alternatively you could simply use a route you have walked previously in 30 minutes and aim to walk beyond the original finish point.

weeks 9–10

Now you should be noticing changes in your fitness and your waistline. You are ready to progress, and introducing uphill and downhill walking is a great way to improve your cardiovascular fitness. Find a hill either in a park or a street, and walk up without stopping. Use the walk back down to get your breath back. You will still be working your muscles, just in a different way! You can make this a 15 minute part of your workout – walking to and from the hill is a good warm-up and cool-down.

weeks 11–12

Another way to progress is to walk while holding weights. These don't have to cost money and can be two tins of beans! Walk your regular routes and focus on your pace and arm swing. To make sure your grip remains strong, secure the weights to your hands or wrists with string or loops of elastic. To have a mixed workout over the week, vary your programme each day – one day with weights, one day with hills and one day on the flat. Keep smiling and walk your way to fitness.

walking and swimming

You can easily combine the swimming and walking programmes:

- Alternate week one of walking with week one of swimming and so on. You may need to repeat weeks so you don't push yourself too much.
- Once you are able to exercise four times a week, it is easy to adapt the programmes to walking twice a week and swimming twice a week and do both!

It really is up to you to choose what you enjoy and what suits you best.

taking it outdoors: running/jogging

Starting to run is just as easy to achieve as the walking programme – it just depends on what you set yourself as a goal. Diabetes doesn't stop you running and if you monitor your insulin requirements as you get fitter you can run as much as you like! All the advice to consider before starting any form of exercise is just as important before starting to run, especially the advice on foot care (see page 86): it's particularly important to wear the right trainers (see page 71).

your running programme

Aim to follow this programme three times a week to see the best results in your fitness.

week 1

Start by walking for five minutes, swinging your arms and keeping up a quick, steady pace. Then jog at an easy pace for one minute. Repeat this four times and to finish add an extra five minute walk to cool down. If you can, persuade a friend to train with you, or failing that get them to be your coach and ask them to time your walks and runs. They will soon be running with you when they see your fitness improving.

week 2

Start by walking for four minutes, then jog for two minutes. Repeat this four times, adding your cool-down walk at the end for five minutes. If you have a dog or can borrow one from a neighbour, they will love the run/walk session and keep you company into the bargain.

week 3

This is the week things really start to change and your runs become longer than your walks! Start by walking for three minutes, then jog for four minutes. Repeat this four times. This is when your timing buddy will really start to wish they had started running when you did, and your neighbour's dog will want a rest!

week 4

Not much walking this week! Start with a two minute walk, then jog for six minutes. Repeat this four times. Now you are jogging for 20 minutes altogether: who would have expected that four weeks ago?

week 5

Walk for two minutes to warm up and then increase your jogging time to eight minutes this week. Repeat three times. Now you are jogging for longer, it's time to focus on your posture. Relax your shoulders, and keep your breathing steady. Try breathing in through your nose and out through your mouth. This will help warm the air before it gets to your lungs and stop your chest from feeling tight.

weeks 6–7

Now you have an established routine of jogging three times a week, it is time to speed things up a little. Introduce swinging your arms and focus on striding out as you jog. See how quickly your jog can become a run once you increase your pace. Many mobile phones now have built-in GPS which will help you monitor your distance, or simply use a route you have jogged previously and aim to run beyond the original finish point. Start by walking for two minutes and then jog/run for 10 minutes. Repeat this three times.

week 8

Congratulations for sticking at your running programme and making it to week eight. Now you should be noticing real changes in your fitness and your waistline! From now on, walk for five minutes at the start and finish of your run to warm up and cool down. Try to jog/run for 20 minutes between your walks for your first two sessions this week and 30 minutes at the end of the week.

Now you have become a runner, aim to run for 30 minutes three times a week. Your fitness and stamina will continue to improve. If you set your goal as running a race for charity, book your place now as you are well on the way to achieving your first five kilometres!

find out more

diabetes
Diabetes UK
www.diabetes.org.uk

American Diabetes Association
www.diabetes.org/

Desmond (diabetes education project)
www.desmond-project.org.uk

Diabetes Education Network
www.diabetes-education.net

Dose Adjustment For Normal Eating
www.dafne.uk.com

NHS Choices
www.nhs.uk

NHS Diabetes
www.diabetes.nhs.uk

Pituitary Foundation (for diabetes insipidus)
www.pituitary.org.uk

healthy lifestyle
Clearing the Air
www.clearingtheairscotland.com (in Scotland)

Eatwell
www.eatwell.gov.uk

GI Diet Guide
www.the-gi-diet.org

Smokefree
www.smokefree.nhs.uk (England and Wales)